A Twentieth Century Fund Book

The Twentieth Century Fund sponsors and supervises timely analyses of economic policy, foreign affairs, and domestic political issues. Not-for-profit and non-partisan, the Fund was founded in 1919 and endowed by Edward A. Filene.

BEYOND
MEDICARE

MALVIN SCHECHTER

with the assistance of
Irma Schechter

BEYOND MEDICARE

Achieving
Long-Term Care
Security

A Twentieth Century Fund Book

Jossey-Bass Publishers · San Francisco

For sales outside the United States, contact Maxwell Macmillan International Publishing Group, 866 Third Avenue, New York, New York 10022.

Manufactured in the United States of America

The paper used in this book is acid-free and meets the State of California requirements for recycled paper (50 percent recycled waste, including 10 percent postconsumer waste), which are the strictest guidelines for recycled paper currently in use in the United States.

10% POST CONSUMER WASTE

The ink in this book is either soy- or vegetable-based and during the printing process emits fewer than half the volatile organic compounds (VOCs) emitted by petroleum-based ink.

Library of Congress Cataloging-in-Publication Data

Schechter, Malvin.
  Beyond medicare : achieving long-term care security / Malvin Schechter, with the assistance of Irma Schechter.
    p.   cm. — (The Jossey-Bass health series)
  Includes bibliographical references and index.
  ISBN 1-55542-583-6
  1. Long-term care of the sick—United States. 2. Long-term care of the sick—United States—Finance. 3. Long-term care of the sick—Government policy—United States. 4. Insurance, Long-term care—United States. I. Schechter, Irma. II. Title. III. Series.
  RA644.6.S34   1993
  362.1'6'0973—dc20   93-14558
                                                                              CIP

Credits are on page 159.

FIRST EDITION
HB Printing   10 9 8 7 6 5 4 3 2 1   *Code 9390*

THE JOSSEY-BASS HEALTH SERIES

CONTENTS

Contents

FOREWORD

Over the last few years, health care has emerged as a major national political issue. The Clinton administration's emphasis on reforming the health care system has heightened the attention to this issue. At the same time, in the areas of employment and economic growth, there is increasing recognition that the aging of our work force has tremendous implications for public and private enterprises alike. These two areas of American life interact directly in the growing problem of long-term health care for America's elderly aged — those who, in ever-increasing numbers, are living to be seventy-five or more.

Long-term care is different from other health care. It is chiefly family and community-based care, supplemented by professional services. The social emphasis of long-term care distinguishes it from acute care, in which the predominant conditions are medical. Long-term health care does not involve just the patient; it makes demands on relatives, friends, and neighbors. But again, altered demographics have changed the picture. American women were once the main source of this sort of health care. But today they are well established as full participants in the work force with their own careers. Families are no longer as geographically connected as in the past, and it is difficult for children to look after parents who live far away. And, in a troubled economy, middle-class families who are ineligible for public assistance are hit the hardest — emotionally as well as financially — as aging relatives begin to need help with the activities of daily life.

Malvin Schechter presents compelling arguments and provocative recommendations for a rational approach to long-term care as part of broad reforms in American health care. He challenges us with the statement that if other nations (and some states) have been successful in reconciling long-term care with acute care services and financing, why aren't we?

Beyond Medicare is one of a group of studies of critical domestic issues that the Twentieth Century Fund has been examining; along with such studies as Bruce Vladeck's *Unloving Care* (1980), Bradford Gray's *The Profit Motive* (1991), the soon-to-be-released book on organ transplants by Jeffrey Prottas, and ongoing studies of access to health care, it marks our determination to enhance the debate on this subject so important to all of us. The Fund thanks Malvin Schechter for his thoughtful and caring approach to this difficult subject.

New York, New York   Richard C. Leone
August 1993   *President*
                                          The Twentieth Century Fund

PREFACE

My father died at age sixty-nine of lung cancer after an operation at the start of his retirement. My mother took care of him at home. Thanks to Medicare coverage of his hospitalizations and physician services, she was saved from impoverishment. Now eighty and in a nursing home after a stroke, she has poor mobility, hand movement, and memory. Medicare paid for her hospitalization but did not cover her outpatient drug costs and long-term care services. The lack of insurance complicated her search for help as she outran her health and wealth. Mom went on Medicaid, impoverished.

My widowed father-in-law, age ninety-two, is in fragile health. His fate — in terms of financial independence and access to competent, organized medical and other professional services — depends on matters he can neither control nor understand. He is not alone in his anxiety over the mysterious discriminations made by our social institutions among people who behaved responsibly throughout their lives and happen to have one disease and its consequences rather than another.

My father, mother, and father-in-law saw the birth of social security and Medicare. They, as well as two subsequent generations of our family, are thankful for these programs. Taken together, however, the programs fall short in an era of chronic illness and longer lifetimes.

Whatever is done — or not done — by government and the private sector to improve financial and service programs for our children or our parents has intergenerational implications. The absence of long-term care affects family members of all ages, emotionally and financially. My wife and I, both in our sixties, have to share our energies and other resources among our parents and our children, and we have to provide for the present and the future. Other families face similar challenges. Lack of well-organized and -financed long-term care is a gap experienced by all too many families. It is the subject of this book.

Purpose of the Book

The main thesis of this book is that long-term care is a necessity in modern America, given life expectancy, growth in the older population, the caregiving demands on young adults as well as older adults, and the stresses on the ever-changing family structure.

While many books offer to show people how to negotiate the barriers to long-term care, *Beyond Medicare* aims at removing the barriers by posing the following questions:

- Instead of each family's struggling to figure out the right course of action — care at home, in the community, or in the nursing home — and then finding and organizing the services, why shouldn't we have reliable, expert service systems standing ready for use?
- Instead of families' paying exorbitantly for services that may not even be the right ones, why not have systems of long-term care that provide the needed expertise and that all can afford?
- If our country can achieve many of these objectives for hospitalization to meet acute care needs, why not for chronic care needs, including long-term care, as well?

Scope

The book presents arguments against attempts to eliminate, delay, or dilute provisions for long-term care. Such attempts derive from concern over the cost of the benefits. Since the package as a whole may require new taxes, proponents of this perspective contend that long-term care is too much for Americans to afford. From another standpoint comes the contention that long-term care costs cannot be controlled and that the technology for delivering long-term care effectively is inadequate. Both these contentions are disputed here.

Beyond Medicare maintains that the time has come for America to care for the young and the old who must live with disability. We must decide on the public and private policies that will generate efficient, equitable, and humane services. To do so, we have to be willing to think afresh. While it is convenient to talk about the country's health care problems in terms of insurance, public assistance, hospitals, and doctors, restricting our thinking to those issues may prove counterproductive. We already see the negative effects of certain policies:

- *Linking health insurance to the job:* the unemployed and their children have no coverage.
- *Programs focused on the poor:* they tend to be underfunded, inadequate, and stigmatizing.
- *Health care that stops short of long-term care in the home and community:* it may result in unnecessary institutionalization, inadequate service, or deterioration in patients' health, leading to the need for acute care.

The following chapters define the problems at hand, point to working programs that resolve those problems and improve the quality of participants' lives, and provide critical reviews of the proposed policies for organizing and financing the delivery of long-term care. I take a novel approach, arguing that long-term care cannot be patterned on the organizational and financial models that exist for acute care. A sound program must emulate geriatric care, which focuses on helping patients function in activities of daily living. The approach is useful not only for geriatric patients but for disabled individuals of all ages.

Timeliness

Although older people stand the greatest risk of needing long-term care, the issue is of vital interest for all Americans, no matter where in the life cycle they find themselves. Members of the middle class are scared that their health insurance is disintegrating. Not only are they afraid of losing their financial protection, but they recognize the potential for financial catastrophe: with no reliable third-party programs to take over the costs of long-term care, individuals who must shoulder that burden run the risk of actual impoverishment. This reality underscores the timeliness of the main topic of this book—health care reform to provide secure long-term care.

Audience

Beyond Medicare was written primarily for the makers of public and private policy at a time when leaders are struggling with issues related to health reform and are looking for essential information on which to base America's new health policies, including security of long-term care. The book should be valuable to leaders in business, philanthropy, and government (from the White House to state capitals); to executives in health care, employee benefits, and social services; to providers of care; and to the general public: consumers and their families.

Contents

Emphasizing the necessity of long-term care in modern America, Chapter One introduces the policy issues and options. The chapter defines long-term care and notes that disabled people of any age may need it but that the elderly are the principal users.

Chapter Two delineates the size of the long-term care problem today and in the future, including the demographic and socioeconomic conditions and the status of service utilization important in formulating policy. Because long-term care involves family members and other "informal caregivers," I consider the implications for changes in family structure and roles. The characteristics of patients and caregivers are also discussed.

Chapter Three explains the nature of geriatrics, professional services geared to people who have or risk having heart disease, stroke, dementia, depression, arthritis, poor vision or hearing or some combination of these. Professional services, in the form of preventive, acute, rehabilitative, mental health, and long-term care, need to be tailored to the individual, after capacities, problems, and life-style have been taken into account. The description of a professional evaluation as the basis for care planning furnishes readers with a standard for making personal decisions. Geriatrics is portrayed as a style of professional practice that integrates a variety of disciplines within medical, mental health, and social services. Despite the growth in the very old population who require a spectrum of care, there is a shortage of trained personnel for chronic care across the board.

Chapter Four depicts several systems that carry out the goals of geriatrics or the goals of chronic care, particularly for those in the frailest condition. Although nursing homes are vital in long-term care for certain kinds of patients, this chapter emphasizes existing systems that provide primary and other care in the community — for despite the unfriendly climate among financial programs attuned to acute care, a few token systems do show us what we otherwise miss in our communities.

Based on these descriptions of professional care and the systems to implement it, Chapters Five and Six critique the major health care financing programs. Chapter Five focuses on Medicaid, Medicare, and Medigap and their deficiencies in providing financial protection, promoting sound care, and reinforcing individual and family self-reliance. Chapter Six looks at private long-term care insurance and questions its credentials with respect to geriatrics, systems support, financial stability, and population coverage.

Chapter Seven reviews major policy options involving long-term care. Chapter Eight offers our recommendations. Long-term care security is pictured as a melding of geriatrics, systems, and social insurance. Medicare in its present form must be transcended for the disabled of all ages who need chronic care. A plan for phasing in such a program and financing it is outlined.

"The cost of long-term care has become the single greatest threat to the financial security of older Americans," the U.S. Senate Special Committee on Aging said in 1985, adding: "The need for long-term care is the last uninsured event of the life cycle." The statement is still true, but that need not be the case much longer.

New York, New York   Malvin Schechter
August 1993

ACKNOWLEDGMENTS

Many people have nourished this book. Our own family has been instructive and supportive: Nathan Cohen, Rose Schechter, Joy Schechter, Daniel James Schechter (a physician assistant), Larry Schechter, and Laura Schechter.

We also owe our professional family many thanks. At the top of the list is Robert N. Butler, chair of the Department of Geriatrics and Adult Development of the Mount Sinai School of Medicine, City University of New York, and director of the International Leadership Center on Longevity and Society (U.S.), the logistics base for much of the work that went into the book.

The wider circle of professional support included staff at the Jewish Home and Hospital for Aged, the Department for the Aging, New York City, and the Miami Jewish Home and Hospital for the Aged at Douglas Gardens, particularly Elliot Stern and Judith Williams.

The staff of the Twentieth Century Fund, especially Carol Kahn, who edited the manuscript, displayed impressive fortitude and judgment. Many kindnesses, including that of vigorous disagreement, were shown to us by Dennis Kodner of Metropolitan Jewish Geriatric Center and Elderplan (in Brooklyn), Joshua M. Wiener of the Brookings Institution (Washington, D.C.), and James P. Firman of the United Seniors Health Cooperative (Washington, D.C.). We learned from the late Representative Claude D. Pepper and his associate Kathryn Gardner-Cravedi,

Samuel Saidin of the Hunter-Brookdale Center on Aging, Judith Feder and Edward Howard, formerly of the Pepper Commission, and officials of the province of Manitoba and the states of Oregon and New York. Basically, this book has been a pop-and-mom operation. We take full parental responsibility for it, with its defects and merits.

                                                              M.S.

                                                              I.S.

THE AUTHORS

Malvin Schechter is a journalist who became a policy analyst and assistant professor of geriatrics and adult development at Mount Sinai School of Medicine, City University of New York. He received his B.A. degree (1952) in history from Columbia University and his M.S. degree (1953) from the Graduate School of Journalism, Columbia University.

In 1959, he received a fellowship from the Ford Foundation to become prepared as a journalist in the field of aging—to cover scientific as well as political, economic, and other issues related to longevity. Schechter has reported on medical and political affairs from Washington for medical and other publications. He covered the enactment and implementation of the Medicare and Medicaid laws as well as developments in biomedicine and health policy during the Johnson, Nixon, Ford, and Carter administrations.

A major interest of Schechter's has been public disclosure of the conduct of government-financed programs like Medicare and Medicaid. In 1972, with the help of Ralph Nader's litigation group, he filed a lawsuit under the Freedom of Information Act to secure records of Medicare inspections of nursing homes. Eventually, the program was required by law to reveal reports on nursing homes, clinical laboratories, hospitals, and physicians.

Schechter has also published newsletters on topics related

to health care and aging. In 1979, he joined the National Institute on Aging as an assistant to the founding director, Robert N. Butler.

In 1982, he accompanied Butler to the Mount Sinai School of Medicine in New York, where he helped to build its department of geriatrics and adult development—the only department of its kind in the 127 medical schools in the United States. Besides being an assistant professor of geriatrics and adult development, Schechter is associate director of the International Leadership Center on Longevity and Society (U.S.), which collaborates with other organizations doing research and education on topics of population aging. Schechter has coauthored *Aging 2000: A Challenge for Health Policy* (1982, with P. Selby), prepared for the 1981 United Nations World Assembly on Aging, and assisted in writing *The Geriatric Patient* (1978, edited by W. Reichel).

Irma Schechter, a freelance writer and consultant in the fields of aging and health, received her B.S. degree (1957) in sociology from Brooklyn College and her M.P.A. degree (1974) in public administration from American University. In her varied career, she has founded two Washington-based newsletters (*Aging Services News* and *Aging Research & Training News*) and written two *Chartbooks on Federal Programs in Aging* (1978, 1981). She has also served as head of the government affairs department of the Visiting Nurse Service of New York, the largest home-health agency in this country. Since 1986, she has written on health and social care issues for senior citizens and lectured abroad on services and personnel training in geriatrics.

BEYOND
MEDICARE

1

Long-Term Care: A Necessity for the Modern Lifespan

Medicare pays for only 45 percent
of older people's health expenses; the balance
must come from their own incomes and savings, or
from Medicaid, which requires a humiliating means test.
A serious illness can mean instant poverty.
—Butler, 1975, p. 4

What is long-term care? It is a combination of health and social services that provide continuing care for the disabled. The purpose of this type of care is to help them live as freely as possible in their customary environment or in the environment that is least restrictive. It is care that continues for an extended period of time to maintain the impaired individual at home, in the community, and in institutions like nursing homes. Long-term care may be relatively simple (involving the help of another person to go to the bathroom, for example) or complex (involving a team of professional, semiprofessional, and laypeople). If the long-term care disappeared, the individual's health and quality of life would deteriorate.

Jumble of Policies, Programs, and Services

Access to long-term care is a necessity of modern life, just as much as access to medical services is. But the United States has no national long-term care policy. It has many half policies, the biggest being "long-term care for anyone who becomes poor and needs a nursing home in a state where there are vacant beds, but do not bother about home care and community-based services (like adult day care), because they are very limited." This is Medicaid.

Private insurance for long-term care is another partial policy, an illusion of protection: too expensive if its protections are worthwhile, and even then, full of caveats and gaps. Medicare, which is public insurance, stops at the door of long-term care but is affected by it.

Long-term care is said to be the last major financial catastrophe of life awaiting some form of insurance (Scanlon, 1990, p. 8). Middle-class individuals and families in need of long-term care are left to improvise an escape from pauperization and Medicaid. State Medicaid officials comment bitterly about middle-class people who hire attorneys to show them how to qualify by sheltering assets from Medicaid, siphoning off funds the officials say ought to go to the poor. But people say they do not want their hard-earned life savings to go for the nursing home. Their equally bitter criticism may be represented by the question, Why are we guarded against pauperization from hospitalization but not from long-term care?

The country's health insurance system needs serious repair. As many companies move to reduce their work forces and fringe benefits, people who have coverage find it is withering. Or they lose it and are exposed to financial catastrophe from health costs. Over thirty-five million Americans are uninsured.

Besides the uninsured, who include working adults and their children, there are millions of other Americans who have inadequate insurance furnished through employment. In hard times, the serious deficiencies of this method of providing access to health services become starkly evident. Other basic problems with the American pattern of health insurance include resistance to paying for preventive medicine and to covering people whose sickness or disability experience mark them as potentially high users of costly services.

With "regular" health insurance under fire because of these

problems, we may question seriously whether it makes sense to go the insurance route in long-term care, a domain in which private insurance has only just gotten started.

The goals of universality, financial security, service availability, and thrift are not only important in regular health care but also in long-term care. These goals may be attained far more effectively and efficiently through an approach closer to social insurance than to private insurance.

To finance a comprehensive long-term care program through social insurance would require every worker to pay a tax of 0.8 percent on wages and every employer to pay the same rate (Rivlin and Wiener, 1988). For example, a $30,000-a-year employee would pay $5 a week and the employer would pay the same to support the program.

This individual might never need long-term care in a nursing home. But in the event of such need, he or she would be spared having to dig into savings and other assets to pay the cost, now often exceeding $40,000 a year. (The individual also would be spared, after savings are exhausted, having to apply for Medicaid.) Moreover, the funds collected from all employers and employees would finance the development and operation of programs of long-term care at home and in the community.

Long-Term Care Reform

President Clinton is committed to achieving major reforms by shoring up the current structure of health insurance. In long-term care, where patchworks substitute for systems, a national framework for financing and for delivering the services has to be created throughout the United States. Long-term care reform is a companion to health care reform. We will make the case later in this book that containment of health care costs requires a strong long-term program.

In making policy for long-term care security, our country's leaders will have to examine problems of organizing services and financing them, particularly the problems that produce a sieve rather than a safety net from private insurance, Medicare, Medicaid, and Medigap. This book explores those problems.

Understanding them is politically important in the crucible of controversies surrounding the deficit; otherwise we may end up being pennywise and pound foolish.

Americans lack long-term care security. In his presidential campaign, Bill Clinton recognized the popularity of the long-term care issue. He promised to expand Medicare into home- and community-based care. (Medicare, it should be noted, applies not only to people at least age sixty-five but also under certain conditions to Americans too disabled to work.) Presented as a benefit for families and people of all ages, long-term care has major vote-getting potential (Exhibit 1.1). Eight in ten voters already have had experience with long-term care problems in obtaining services and paying for them.

As president supported by the Democratic-led Congress, Clinton has the opportunity to set this country on a course of

Exhibit 1.1. Registered Voters' Views on Long-Term Care.

Most American adults have had direct experience with long-term care and are sensitive to the financial and emotional costs. Recent surveys of registered voters produce these views on long-term care:

- One-half understood that Medicare covers little to none of long-term care costs.
- There was a recognition of the need for long-term care insurance, particularly if administered by states rather than the federal government or privately.
- By a ratio of nearly two to one, middle-aged and older Americans preferred a social insurance program to one based on private financing with a government subsidy for the poor.
- Nearly seven in ten voters said they would pay more taxes specifically for a government program covering long-term care.
- Long-term care was consistently cited as the top priority for government spending against all other issues.
- Nine of ten voters believe it would be financially devastating for most working and middle-income families to have a member needing long-term care; most said they could not afford long-term care costs—even those with incomes of $50,000.
- By five to one, they agreed that a long-term program should cover all ages, not just the elderly.
- One out of four of those polled stated it was "morally wrong" to place aging parents in a nursing home rather than have them live with the family.
- Older people worry about catastrophic illness.
- The polls showed a clear preference for home care over nursing home care.

Source: Adapted from McConnell, 1988.

universal coverage and comprehensive benefits, including long-term care. The fact that the legislative process for broad reforms of health care begins with a kernel of long-term care is no guarantee that long-term care will be in it at the end—or in it adequately. Much will depend on what the president and the Congress hear from the American people, and that in turn depends on their knowledge and goals.

The translation of Clinton's proposal for home care into law is a long-awaited event. His predecessors preferred not to move beyond Medicare's original borders. In 1988, Congress enacted, then repealed, a Medicare Catastrophic Coverage Act with major new benefits but not long-term care. Among justifications for holding back on long-term care was that the time was not right, given the rapid inflation in conventional Medicare costs.

Now, we have a president who makes the case that health costs in general, not only Medicare, must be controlled as an essential part of deficit reduction and national economic growth. At the same time, he has spoken of investment in the nation's human resources and infrastructure. He has asked the nation to reduce costs and invest simultaneously. If Congress can be persuaded that long-term care is an essential part of the investment and health-cost control, the days of delay—hardly unimportant to eighty- and ninety-year-olds and their families—will be over.

Interrelationship of Reforms

Long-term care reform is an essential component of health care reform. Discussions of cost containment in health care cannot be confined to acute care only. The division in the financing and organization of services between acute and long-term care has become a harmful artifice at a time when the leading health problems of America are chronic illnesses. It is an artifice sanctioned by our institutions, allotting to private insurance the coverage of most workers and dependents and to philanthropy and government the coverage of the poor, the mentally and physically disabled who cannot work or represent too high a risk for insurance, and the retired.

Just as attempts to squeeze a balloon in one place will make it expand in another, economies in the acute care sector will be nullified by cost shifts into long-term care, and vice versa. Likewise, ceilings on government payments to hospitals and doctors are nullified by cost shifts into private insurance. The game benefits some players and will continue to be played until the public focuses on the total picture and tells its leaders to change the rules. Because of the effect on Medicaid, state governments and people with chronic illness who are impoverished have a vital stake in the national health care reforms that Congress and the White House bring about. Those who face future impoverishment from care expenses also have a stake in all this — a Sword of Damocles that hangs above all but the very wealthy.

Policy decisions about long-term care will occur within the framework of strategies to spur the economy, reduce the federal deficit, and control inflation in doctor and hospital expenses. While one might argue that today is not the time for long-term care initiatives, especially if they require major new government spending, long-term care spending will rise even without new policies. The major reason is demographics.

Turning from How Much to How Many

An estimated eleven million Americans, old and young, need long-term care. Two-thirds are elders and one-third are children and adults under age sixty-five, including persons with acquired immune deficiency (AIDS), cerebral palsy, and other chronic illnesses. All need access to a balanced system of institutional and noninstitutional services to promote their ability to function. The fastest-growing population segment is the group aged eighty-five and older, now about three million and destined to almost triple by 2030 (Figure 1.1). Meanwhile, the baby-boom cohort born between 1946 and 1964 is moving toward retirement. The combination of a huge cohort and the improvement in life expectancy after age sixty-five poses policy issues that cannot be put off safely. (See Chapter Two for more discussion of demographics.)

Figure 1.1. U.S. Population, by Age and Gender, 1989 and 2030.

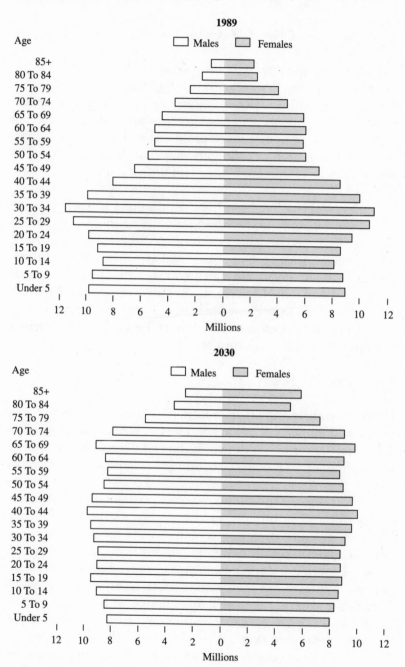

Source: U.S. Bureau of the Census, 1989, 1990a.

A Rising Tide of Very Old Americans

Thanks to progress in medicine, public health, and general living standards, most Americans reach old age, and many reach very old age. This is when long-term care and its financing become a major worry. The average American has a 16 percent chance of having one or more problems with activities of daily living (ADLs), such as eating and bathing, by age eighty. The figure rises to 44 percent by age eighty-five (Institute of Medicine, 1985).

Most elders live their lives without major losses of functional ability from the diseases and other conditions for which long-term care is needed, such as heart disease, cancer, stroke, Alzheimer's disease, osteoporosis, and arthritis. Almost 80 percent of them will spend less than $5,000 in their lifetimes on long-term care, and only 13 percent will spend more than $40,000. But people can never know for sure that they will be in the fortunate majority to escape hardship. (Chapter Three describes geriatrics and the geriatric patient.)

What Families Do

Family members and other "informal" or unpaid caregivers provide about 80 percent of long-term care. Government, private insurance, and the health professions all depend on the ability and willingness of families to continue being pillars of long-term care.

The American family, however, is changing in size and composition. The number of women caregivers and the time they can give are declining. For the first time in history, the average married couple has more parents than children. Future middle-generation women can expect to spend more years with parents over sixty-five than with children under eighteen. More women are entering the work force than ever before, and they are tending to work longer, creating an increasing demand for "outside" assistance. Yet at the same time, the government is struggling to curb costs and limit the use of nursing homes by introducing or expanding home and community-based care. The effort is inadequate; it falls short of reaching those individuals whose needs are not (yet) at the nursing home level.

AIDS and Aging

Competition for America's limited long-term care services is under way between people with acquired immune deficiency syndrome (AIDS) and older people. Through new therapies, including drugs, AIDS has become a prolonged disease. Patients are getting older, some return to their parents' or other relatives' homes, and among their caregivers are older people. Much of what has been learned about care in nursing homes, home care, hospice care, and other long-term care for the frail elderly can be applied to people with AIDS, some of whom are covered by Medicaid. In short, AIDS and aging issues are intertwined (Riley, Ory, and Zablotsky, 1989).

State Activity in Long-Term Care

Some 250 state and federal programs offer long-term care in the form of personal assistance services, mainly through attendants and homemakers. In 1988, these services covered over two million persons, or only 26 percent of noninstitutionalized Americans estimated to need such help. The cost was $3.4 billion, with each program shaped by available funding and state and local priorities.

Public funding sources include the following: Medicaid, through its waiver programs for home and community care and its personal care option program; Social Services Block Grants (SSBG); Title III of the Older Americans Act; the Aid and Attendants Allowance under the Department of Veterans Affairs; Vocational Rehabilitation Act; Medicare; and state-only programs.

A pacesetter in home and community services, the Medicaid waiver programs provide an alternative to nursing homes mostly for severely disabled people. In 1987, some 76,000 elderly and disabled persons received this help. The Medicaid personal care option and SSBG programs served 264,000 and

877,920 clients, respectively, in 1988. Title III, in serving 701,220 clients, offered only a few hours of care to people with lesser needs (Simon-Rusinowitz, 1991).

These community-based long-term care services tend to have weak connections with medical and hospital systems. This has been overcome in scattered projects (discussed in Chapter Four) that provide for the continuing care — including various health and social services — needed by frail and disabled people. These small continuing care systems demonstrate practical technologies for comprehensive assistance to disabled persons. The funding to create more of these systems is eagerly awaited.

Problems States Face

All fifty states have problems in the delivery of long-term care services. The scattering of elders in rural states and their concentration in highly urban states make for variations on common themes in finding and serving people who need help. Many older people are both frail and poor. Multicultural and multiracial areas pose particular challenges in developing effective services. In 1990, about 89 percent of elders were white, 8 percent were black, and about 3 percent other races (including American Indian, Eskimo, Aleut, and Asian and Pacific Islanders). Persons of Hispanic origin may be of any race; they make up 4 percent of the elderly.

The heaviest burden of meeting long-term care needs is found in nine states. About half the nation's elders live in California (three million); Florida and New York (two million plus each); and Pennsylvania, Texas, Illinois, Ohio, Michigan, and New Jersey (one million each). (The map in Figure 1.2 shows the national distribution.)

In 1986, the National Governors' Association adopted an enlightened statement calling for the development of continuing care systems. Individuals and families would have an identifiable place in the community to go for information, evaluation of needs, care planning, and care coordination. The governors recommended pooling Medicaid and Medicare funding to support systems to unite acute and long-term care.

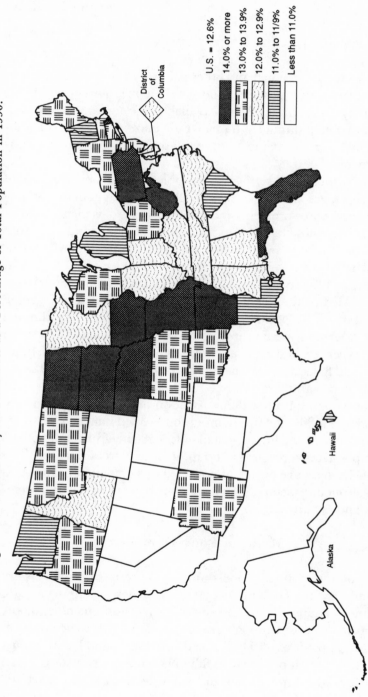

Figure 1.2. Persons Sixty-Five and Over as a Percentage of Total Population in 1990.

District
of
Columbia

U.S. = 12.6%

14.0% or more

13.0% to 13.9%

12.0% to 12.9%

11.0% to 11/9%

Less than 11.0%

Hawaii

Alaska

Source: Program Resources Department, American Association of Retired Persons, and U.S. Administration on Aging, 1991, pp. 6–7 (based on data from the U.S. Bureau of the Census).

Missing Elements

Important professional and other paid services—like home care, social supportive services, and geriatric medicine—are absent in many communities. When available, they are uncoordinated, hard to obtain through a bureaucratic maze, likely to be of questionable quality, and expensive relative to individual and family income.

Institutional services are problematic as well. Because of bed shortages, nursing homes are choosy about patients, preferring those whose problems and costs are more convenient or profitable. Unlike hospitals, nursing homes are predominantly for-profit institutions; they are reluctant to take patients under the principal organized payer of long-term care, the federal-state Medicaid program. Quality of care in nursing homes is a continuing issue.

Meanwhile, the bill for those who pay the nursing home out of their own pockets averages $35,000 a year. An estimated 500,000 Americans a year slip into poverty because of long-term care expenses, and some apply for Medicaid. At the same time, state and federal governments confront deficits and popular opposition to tax increases.

Except for a few demonstration projects, long-term care programs follow the fragmented sources of finance. They have been designed and implemented independently from one another. The predictable result is overlap, gap, and cross-purpose. The inefficiencies have been compounded by population growth and socioeconomic factors; they have gone beyond patchwork remedies and require basic reforms.

Myths of Long-Term Care

Feeding into political opposition to long-term care reforms are certain myths. To combat them, advocates of long-term care will need support from all ranks of voters—in business, labor, minority groups, women's groups, professionals in health care, and organizations of the disabled. Insurance and health industry groups are more likely to fall in line if they see strong White House leadership, as they did when Medicare was enacted.

Myth 1: Home Care Is Trivial

The first myth involves the mistaken notion that long-term care is trivial. The services are scorned as "baby-sitting" and "maid service," although they are life preserving in a different way from hospital and doctor services.

Part of the disparagement of long-term care may be prejudice against the elderly and others who are disabled and frail. In a production- and youth-oriented society, it may reflect an infatuation with highly sophisticated technology and the drama of acute care medicine. Sexism may also be involved. Long-term care may not look impressive to some when it is provided by women, as relatives of the patient and as paid home care workers. But long-term care is as genuine a response to human need as is acute care represented by physicians, chiefly men.

Myth 2: Families Will Abandon Their Elders

Another myth is that families are waiting eagerly to abandon their elders to paid caregivers. The professional literature and experience with programs in other countries like Canada show that families tend to exhaust themsleves before applying for outside help. When such professionally guided help is provided, family burnout is prevented and members continue to give support commensurate with their abilities.

Myth 3: Long-Term Care Involves Unjustified Demands

There is a fear that a program of insured long-term care would have a "woodwork" effect. This ungracious term suggests that people who do not need services would demand them: like termites, they would surface from the woodwork to get their gratuitous sweets.

There is evidence that America's chronically ill are now underserved. A program that induces them to seek help is hardly a waste and may make the best sense from a public health point of view. In the insurance field, such encouragement might be deplored as raising "loss ratios," or the ratio of benefits paid (the losses, to insurers) to premiums collected. If the "woodwork" myth represents distress with the prospect of having to raise money to meet needs appropriately, discussion should turn directly to that.

The challenge is to separate people with unmet need from those with unjustified demands. Access and cost control issues — which are focused on in general health reform — are equally important in long-term care. Means exist to measure the disability levels and translate them into needs for formal (skilled, paid) services and informal (unpaid, family or volunteer) services. Systems exist in which the use of long-term care services is controlled in line with prescribed budgets.

However, since long-term care in the home and community depend so much on family cooperation, some costs of long-term care should be reserved for encouraging the participation and gaining the cooperation of these caregivers and protecting them against sickness, demoralization, and burnout. Their role in planning care is essential. Respite care is a "support the supporters" benefit by allowing the caregiver time off for a vacation, earning at a temporary job, or attending to personal needs.

Myth 4: Long-Term Care Is Too Expensive

In a trillion-dollar health care economy, with hospitals accounting for 33 percent, long-term care at about 10 percent is a relatively minor expense. Nursing home care far outweighs community and home care as a long-term care expense, by a ratio of about three to one. In acute care, the per patient expense is high and the duration of service short; in long-term care, the reverse is true. As in acute care, there is good reason to invest in research on effective and efficient ways to prevent illness and complications, to treat and rehabilitate patients to slow down or avoid further deterioration, and to organize services and deliver services in ways that stretch the budget.

Most home and community-based services do not require massive investments in highly trained experts, sophisticated machinery, and complex buildings. Long-term care often is labor intensive, but often the labor is without cost to a program (for example, when provided by family members and volunteers) or is relatively low cost (when offered by nurses, aides, and homemakers). A long-term care program can be expanded relatively rapidly.

Any White House policy on long-term care will run a gauntlet through Congress: some will say it is a frill deserving a low priority, that the nation cannot afford it until the uninsured population gets regular health insurance and overall health costs are controlled, that private long-term care insurance should be given a chance before government moves in, and that too little is known about the organization and financing of long-term care.

Without the inclusion of long-term care, however, the architecture of comprehensive health care reform will be seriously flawed. Moreover, demographics and disease are forcing this country to make long-term care policy. Even with no change in policy, spending more money on long-term care is inevitable: this year, next year, and into the future, more and more Americans are going to need long-term care. Outrunning their health, they will outrun their wealth, triggering massive expenditures through Medicaid.

Consider: The very old population is growing rapidly now. A dramatic surge will occur early in the next century. The leading edge of our seventy-six-million baby-boom cohort reaches age sixty-five in the year 2011. The biggest bunch of babies, an enormous electorate, will become the biggest bunch of retirees. Ten years later, they enter the ages of heightened need for long-term care, whether in the community or in nursing homes. Meanwhile, an AIDS epidemic adds to the stress on our patchworks of long-term care.

Looking Ahead

The title of this book, *Beyond Medicare: Achieving Long-Term Care Security,* implies the conditions that will shape our later lives. "Medicare" is emblematic of the public and private sectors' lopsided emphasis on acute care. "Security" is an intended reference to the social security program.

This book argues for basing policy for long-term care on
the social security program, a further evolution of the securi-
ties that began in 1935. The same legislation of the Great Depression that established unemployment insurance and maternal and
child health grants to the states also established monthly cash
benefits for contributors who retire. In 1939, the program expanded to cover the spouse and child survivors of a deceased
worker. In 1950, it expanded to cover disabled workers and dependents. In 1965, it expanded with Medicare, which protects
retirees and disabled workers against the costs of medical and
hospital care.

A strong case can be made that now is the time for social
security to cover long-term care. The principles for long-term
care security are the following:

1. Benefits available universally — to young and old — according
    to need
2. Benefits designed according to principles of geriatrics and
    chronic care, reaching across customary insurance bound-
    aries to unite preventive, acute, and long-term care and
    to cover health and social services in ways appropriate to
    stage of the life cycle
3. Benefits delivered systematically, developed with profes-
    sional and consumer input
4. Benefits financed primarily by payments out of income
    across the working life and by other taxes, such as taxes
    on estates and gifts

We cannot expect these principles to be implemented overnight. Medicare was in operation six months after enactment
because an infrastructure of hospitals and trained personnel was
already in existence. But comprehensive long-term care in a variety of forms adapted to the populations served has to be designed and built in most areas of the country. The organization
and financing of services have to proceed in step. This will not
happen without a commitment to long-term care that stands up
against efforts to bargain it away.

The development of a national program can be staged to coincide with the restoration of the U.S. economy while contributing to the productivity of the families who benefit from organized long-term care. But nothing will happen without a vision supplied by the White House and a commitment of Congress to a practical timetable for achieving that vision. The place of this book in that process is to offer concepts and evidence about comprehensive long-term care. The paths to this goal may be shorter, less fearsome, and more appealing than the reader may imagine.

2

Who Needs and Who Cares: Characteristics of Patients and Caregivers

There are now many more persons
suffering from conditions
that are managed rather than cured.
These conditions may afflict them for decades.
—Rice, 1985, p. 6

A large population at risk of needing long-term care in old age did not appear overnight. Between 1900 and 1990, as America's population more than doubled, the older segment of the population grew eightfold. In 1900, only 4 percent of about 90 million Americans was age sixty-five or more. Today, in an America of 250 million people, the percentage is 12.5. More Americans reach age eighty today than made it to age sixty-five in 1900.

Of every 100 babies born today, 70 are likely to live beyond age sixty-five (Brody and Persky, 1990). The chances are best for white children in richer, more educated families and worst for minority-group children in poor, less educated families.

This chapter provides the statistics on questions of which individuals need care and who cares for them. We will look at the health, demographic, socioeconomic, and other characteristics of patients and caregivers.

18

Who Are the Disabled?

As many as 11 million Americans are disabled enough to need the help of others in basic ADLs. About 4 million are so severely disabled that they require substantial help just to survive; this group includes about 3.3 million elders and 800,000 persons under age sixty-five. (These numbers are difficult to arrive at precisely because of differences in survey methods.)

Perhaps surprising considering their precarious conditions, only 1.5 of these 4.1 million severely disabled persons are in institutions like nursing homes. The United States has 18,000 nursing homes. Some serve multiple purposes, such as short-term rehabilitation and maintenance care (often after a period of hospitalization) and long-term maintenance (or custodial) care.

Americans reaching age sixty-five in a given year have a 43 percent chance of experiencing a nursing home stay of short or long duration at some time during the rest of their lives. Of 2.2 million persons reaching age sixty-five, nearly 1 million will have at least one nursing home stay. Among them, 300,000 will be in a nursing home for at least three months, 223,000 for at least a year, and 85,000 for five or more years (Kemper and Murtaugh, 1991). The proportion of persons institutionalized rises with age — 15 percent between ages sixty-five and seventy-four compared to 21 percent at age eighty-five and older.

The average nursing home resident is a white widow, age eighty, with several chronic conditions or deficiencies in ADLs. She has been in the facility for eighteen months, admitted from a hospital or other facility rather than from her own home. In the next century, more residents are expected from minority populations. Racially and ethnically, long-term care users will resemble the U.S. population mix.

Chronic Conditions and Functional Loss

The rising chances of needing long-term care in late life reflect diseases and other conditions whose rates and severity increase with age (Figure 2.1). Arthritis, hypertension, heart disease,

Figure 2.1. Top Ten Chronic Conditions for
People Sixty-Five and Over, 1989.

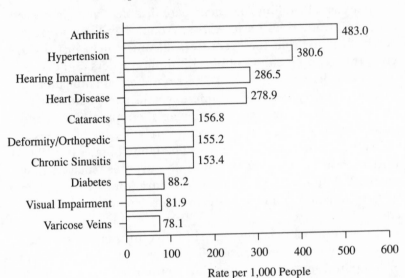

Rate per 1,000 People

Source: National Center for Health Statistics, 1990.

hearing and vision problems, depression, and other chronic conditions become more common with age and occur in combination. This makes medical care more complex. As we will see
in the next chapter, geriatric medicine has to balance competing vulnerabilities or risks in an effort to preserve the patient's
abilities to function, or self-reliance.

For instance, osteoporosis, or bone thinning, is a cause
of 1.2 million fractures a year, and these individuals (chiefly
women) have residual losses of function. Dementia of the Alzheimer type, which affects more than two million people, is believed to affect 3 to 9 percent of all persons age sixty-five and
older and 32 percent of everyone over eighty-five.

Care in the Community

The quality of life or even survival of such disabled people outside of institutions often depends on their living arrangements
(Table 2.1). About half the severely disabled elders live with

Table 2.1. Living Arrangements of Older People, by Age and Gender, March 1989 (Excludes People in Institutions).

Living arrangement	65+		65 to 74		75 to 84		85+	
	Men	*Women*	*Men*	*Women*	*Men*	*Women*	*Men*	*Women*
Total (thousands)	12,078	16,944	7,880	9,867	3,506	5,669	693	1,408
Percent	100.0	100.0	100.0	100.0	100.0	100.0	100.0	100.0
Living with spouse	74.3	40.1	78.4	51.4	70.4	28.1	48.2	9.1
Living with other relatives	7.7	16.9	6.4	13.5	8.7	19.1	17.3	32.6
Living alone	15.9	40.9	13.3	33.5	18.4	50.5	32.6	54.0
Living with nonrelatives	2.1	2.0	2.0	1.5	2.5	2.3	1.7	4.3

Source: U.S. Bureau of the Census, 1990b.

a spouse (one-sixth being poor), about one-third live with someone other than a spouse (almost 59 percent being poor), and
about one-sixth live alone (55.7 percent being poor). This last
group is primarily widows. Because women outlive men, the
problems of very old age and severe disability are problems faced
overwhelmingly by women.

Networks: Formal and Informal

Only 20 percent of long-term care in the community is provided
by the "formal network" of professional and other paid caregivers.
The "informal network" of family members, neighbors, and
volunteers — an estimated 2.2 million caregivers age fourteen
and above in 1982 — aided 1.2 million elders in the community
(Stone, Cafferata, and Sangl, 1986, p. 3). The kind of help given
by caregivers includes shopping, transportation, personal hy-
giene assistance, household tasks, administering medications,
and handling finances.

   Caregivers themselves often are in or approaching old age.
Nearly 50 percent of caregivers are forty-five to sixty-four and 30
percent are sixty-five and over, including 3 percent who are over
seventy-five. Young elders help sustain the older elderly (Stone,
Cafferata, and Sangl, 1986). Wives, daughters, and other women
make up 72 percent of the caregivers (Public Policy Institute,
American Association of Retired Persons, 1989). Middle-aged
women who have caregiving responsibilities for their children
and their parents have been described as a "sandwich generation."

   Given the fact that women live seven years longer than
men on average, it is not surprising that 37 percent of disabled
elderly men are cared for by their wives but only 10 percent
of disabled women are looked after by their husbands (Figure
2.2). Deteriorating health often is a cue for an elder (without
a spouse to rely on) to move in with a son or daughter. These
adult children often have to manage caregiving in addition to
a regular job, and one in seven stop working in order to give
care.

   As age increases, the role of spouse support decreases and
other family members step in to help, women still predominating.

Figure 2.2. Caregivers and Their
Relationship to the Elderly Care Recipient, 1982.

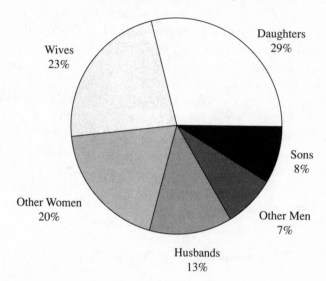

Note: Caregiver population includes primary and secondary caregivers.
Source: Select Committee on Aging, 1987.

An Informal Caregivers Survey (Select Committee on Aging, 1987) found that one-fourth of aging fathers and one-third of aging mothers were cared for by their children. Older women often lack a spouse-caregiver and live alone, increasing their risk of institutionalization if they become ill.

Living Alone as a Risk Factor

About one-third of the elderly population lives alone. In 1985, for the first time, more American women over seventy-five were living alone than in family households. There is a high correlation between living alone and poverty. More than two-thirds of all elders in poverty live alone. Death of a husband may produce poverty because of medical and funeral expenses and lost pension income (Moloney, 1987).

Living alone does not mean total isolation from family. Most older people keep in touch with their families. Over half the elderly in their own households live within thirty minutes of a child, and only 13 percent of elders are more than an hour away from a child. Daily contact with a child by telephone or in person is reported by 41 percent of elders (Public Policy Institute, American Association of Retired Persons, 1989). The proximity permits family members to be of help with personal care and maintaining a household.

Where there is no family or substitute in the community or where the family cannot carry on further, the costs of care go up. Family inadequacy is a risk factor for nursing home use. At an average of $35,000 a year in 1991, the nursing home is where the heaviest per capita expenses and the preponderance of long-term care costs are incurred. About $48 billion of the nation's $60 billion annual bill for long-term care is paid in nursing homes.

Defining Who Needs Help

In recent years, 2.2 million people annually reached age sixty-five, and 1.5 million elders died. This yielded a net addition of 645,000 to an elder population of about 31 million in 1990, about 10 percent being eighty-five and older (including 61,000 centenarians). There were 9.8 million age seventy-five to eighty-four and 18.2 million age sixty-five to seventy-four. These groups have grown, respectively, twenty-four, thirteen, and eight times their size in 1900. About 40 percent of the elderly population is older than seventy-five—the main age category for which long-term care is needed. At age sixty-five, one person in sixteen needs help with at least one ADL. At age eighty-five, one in two needs such help.

A scale based on ability to perform ADLs is used to categorize individuals. The five ADLs are eating, dressing, transferring to and from bed or chair, going to the bathroom, and bathing. Of community-living individuals with such limitations, almost 40 percent have three or more (Public Policy Institute, American Association of Retired Persons, 1989, pp. 32–33). Cognitive and physical impairments often occur together. Almost three-quarters of those with severe cognitive impairment have deficiencies in three or more ADLs. Almost everyone with four or five deficiencies has a group of problems: getting in and out of bed (transferring), dressing, and bathing. A large proportion also have toileting problems. Over 60 percent of nursing home residents have problems with memory or thinking, principally ascribed to Alzheimer's disease.

Chronic illness makes elders the heaviest users of health services. The older the patient, the greater the use of services in every category (except for dental visits). Elders use the hospital twice as often, stay longer, and use twice the prescribed drugs as do younger persons (Special Committee on Aging, U.S. Senate, 1988, p. 37).

Although elders represent 12 percent of the population, they account for 40 percent of all hospital days of care. The 4 percent of the population who are over seventy-five account for 15.1 percent of all hospital days. In some cases, the hospital stay is prolonged while attempts are made to place the patient for convalescence and long-term care in a home care program or a nursing home (Public Policy Institute, American Association of Retired Persons, 1989).

Not only is there more use of hospitals and doctors but also — often for the first time in most people's lives — the use of nursing homes, home health agencies, and social services. As the very old population expands, their aggregate demand for hospital services will grow and expenses will increase.

For example, the risk of hip fracture rises exponentially with age. One in five women who have a hip fracture dies in the first year afterward, and another one in five loses the ability to walk unaided. Estimating only acute hospitalization costs and surgeons' fees (nursing home and home care costs not being available), the number of hip fractures — 220,000 in 1987 — is expected to reach 300,000 in 2000; the costs would rise to $2 billion from $1.6 billion in constant 1987 dollars. By 2040, the projection is between 530,000 and 840,000 hip fractures a year at an annual cost of $6 billion (Schneider and Guralnik, 1990).

Functional limitations raise the chances of needing hospital and doctor care. Some 42 percent of persons with severe limitations have one or two hospitalizations a year — three times the rate for unimpaired elders. A severely impaired person (having at least three ADL deficiencies) averages twelve doctor visits a year, while most elders make about four. Elders are relatively heavy users of home health services, prescribed drugs, over-the-counter drugs, vision and hearing aids, and medical equipment and supplies.

Health Care Expenses

No wonder, then, that elders account for one-third of the nation's annual spending for personal health care, although they comprise one-eighth of the population. The estimate for total national spending in 1990 was nearly $666 billion, about $220 billion being for elders. Nursing home care was $53 billion. Medically related home health care was $8.5 billion, and other home care was an unspecified amount in an $11.3 billion category of "other personal health care," which included some Medicaid funds for home and community-based services (Levit, Lazenby, Cowan, and Letsch, 1991).

Spending Increases

The volume of health care services per capita is growing for the nation as a whole, partly because the elder population is expanding. For the chief components of health care spending—hospital and doctor care—the trend has been more services per capita, with each unit of service becoming more costly. For the principal payers of health services for the elderly (Medicare and Medicaid), trends in prices, intensity of services, and population growth seem to offer no respite. While the elder population grew relatively little between 1977 and 1984, their personal health care spending virtually tripled in this period (to $120 billion from $43 billion).

In the late 1980s, following liberalizations in Medicare and Medicaid, spending for home health care grew rapidly. Spending in 1990 was 22.1 percent over 1989, in turn 24.9 percent over the previous year. These were the highest rates of growth in any category of national health spending, which does

not include non–medically determined personal care. Public
sources financed three-quarters of these expenses, and out-of-
pocket spending covered 12 percent. Public programs cover two-
thirds of personal health care spending for elders, including home
health care expense. Medicare alone pays 45 percent of their
total health bill, Medicaid 12 percent, and other government
sources, including the Department of Veterans Affairs, 6 percent.

More Dollars Coming Out of Pocket

Since elders pay 29 percent of their health care expenses out
of pocket, health care inflation threatens their financial condition. Those with the heaviest impairment loads make the highest
out-of-pocket payments. Some of the threat is due to coinsurance
and deductibles required by Medicare and to premiums for supplementary private insurance. But some is due to costs Medicare does not cover, such as long-term nursing home care, which
accounted for 42 percent of 1984 out-of-pocket spending. For
1984, the proportion of out-of-pocket costs taken by hospitals
was 6 percent and by physicians, 21 percent. These are insured
services, whereas nursing home care is virtually uninsured. The
fact that physicians may bill beyond amounts Medicare approves
for payment accounts for the higher uncovered percentage in
contrast to hospitals (Waldo and Lazenby, 1984).

Medicare was the only protection for 20 percent of the
elderly, or five million persons, in 1984. These elders tended
to have low incomes and to have the greatest health care needs
(General Accounting Office, 1992). They also tended to be the
oldest. Even though very old persons have the higher sickness
risks, they were less likely to have private supplementary insurance coverage, or Medigap.

As a group, elders are abnormally sensitive to health care
costs despite government programs. Most of these costs are covered by "insurance" (chiefly Medicare and private supplementary policies) and Medicaid. Out-of-pocket spending by the
elderly is for uninsured services, for the deductibles and copayments required by insurance, for bills exceeding insurance limits
(such as doctor fees above Medicare approved limits), and for

premiums for insurance. All told, 18 percent of elders' incomes is spent on health services, versus 3 percent for nonelders.

Of all out-of-pocket health costs for the elderly, hospital care represented 6 percent, doctor services 21 percent, and nursing home care 42 percent (Waldo and Lazenby, 1984). The proportion of nursing home care paid by patients directly was 51 percent and by Medicaid 42 percent in 1986. Medicare and private insurance together accounted for 2.4 percent (Varner, 1987).

Nursing home costs were not only the largest component of uninsured service for elders but also one of the most inflationary, growing at double-digit rates in the 1970s and 1980s. The average bill for a year in a nursing home in the mid 1980s was $22,000, ranging from $12,000 to $50,000. According to the U.S. Senate aging committee, "The cost at even the lower end of this range is beyond the resources of most older Americans" (Special Committee on Aging, U.S. Senate, 1988, p. 37). Many elders enter the nursing home in poverty or at the brink after having spent heavily for uninsured services at home. Soon after entry, many elders become eligible for Medicaid. According to one study, between one-quarter and two-thirds of private-pay entrants are estimated to become Medicaid clients (Special Committee on Aging, U.S. Senate, 1988, p. 37). Another study estimates that 11 percent convert to Medicaid in the nursing home.

Precision is lacking about the Medicaid spend-down pattern. Conclusions are based on inferences from official data, which do not directly relate the phenomenon to its causes. A high percentage of nursing home users die or go home after brief stays. It is speculated that some long-stay patients remain in private-pay status because they sell their homes. Home care and outpatient drug expenses bring many elders to the door of the nursing home already impoverished (Doty, Liu, Manton, and Harahan, 1989).

Worry about uncovered expenses drives many elders to buy Medigap policies at high expense relative to income, such as $600 a year for a Blue Cross policy. Because of low incomes and because of their relatively high illness risk, the very old are less likely to have insurance in addition to Medicare. Ironically, they may be most in need of conventional coverage as well as protection against long-term care expenses.

Planning for the Future

The foregoing issues will soon be magnified. America of the twenty-first century will have an unprecedentedly large elderly population, not only because average life expectancy will grow but also because the seventy-six-million-member baby-boom population will reach age sixty-five starting in 2011. The American elderly population is expected to almost double to sixty-eight million by 2050, when average life expectancy will reach eighty.

Up: The Very Old Population

Growing faster than the elder population in general, the very old subgroup (eighty-five and older)—the disability-prone subgroup—will grow faster and make up, not one in eight elders, but one in four elders by 2050.

Between now and 2050, events may change the trends and issues. Better understanding of age-related diseases and disabilities through scientific research may reduce rates of disease and disability. Healthier behaviors in early and middle life may produce successive cohorts of healthier elders, hopefully to have fewer years of disability in very old age.

For today, the challenges of meeting long-term care needs are themselves sobering. Currently, a declining trend in death rates has not been accompanied by a change in morbidity or disability rates. If this pattern continues, the United States will have a larger elderly population containing a greater disabled population. For the average American, the better the chances of reaching very old age, the greater the chances of needing long-term care. Baby boomers, whose numbers have stressed the institutions serving childhood through middle age, will also stress the institutions serving old age. Estimates may vary, but the direction is clear. For instance, the disabled elderly population in 2020, when the oldest baby boomers verge on age seventy-five, may range from between ten and fourteen million. Over the next decades, the number may reach as high as twenty-four million.

The projections depend on how disability is defined and assumptions about the future prevalence of disability. The most optimistic scenario has the duration of disability compressed into a smaller part of old age. If disability rates declined as fast as mortality rates, there would be 20 percent fewer disabled elders in 2020 and 30 percent fewer in 2060.

We can hope for cures and preventives for these conditions that will reduce the need for long-term as well as acute care. Possibly methods will be developed and applied to produce a life with no disability until the smallest period before death in old age. But epidemiologic evidence points the other way: for each functionally active year gained in life expectancy, about 3.5 functionally compromised years have been added. The possibility of compressing morbidity into fewer years may be realized by individuals who have good medical care throughout their lives and are able to adopt healthy life-styles and live in nontoxic environments. Generally, these are individuals at higher socioeconomic levels, and this is where the chief gains in disability-free life expectancy are observed.

Up: Nursing Home Use

The Brookings Institution estimates that the number of elders using nursing homes will grow by 76 percent in the next thirty years, faster than the growth of the elder population in the same period (61 percent). In 2018, there may be 4 million. In the same period, the number of elder users of paid home care may rise by 60 percent to nearly 6.5 million (Rivlin and Wiener, 1988). Reasons for such an increase are (1) fewer caregiving children due to lower birth rates after the baby boom ended in 1964, (2) the trend toward living alone, and (3) higher employment rates of women — in the past the main caregivers for the elderly at home.

Delivering the current level of service to elders in 2040 would require doubling the number of home health aides to 484,000. If the current level of service changed substantially, the number of aides might exceed 1.3 million in 2040. What circumstances could make for such a change? The General Accounting Office (1991) described estimates as chancy because the situation is dynamic: "More providers are marketing services, more public programs are financing home care, and more families are willing to purchase home care."

Up: Long-Term Care Costs

The trends and conjectures cited above lead to the conclusion that the nation will see enormous growth in the costs of long-term care. Estimating the cost of nursing home and home care services for elders in 1988 at about $42 billion, the Brookings Institution projected costs to reach $120 billion (in the same dollars) in 2018 and $350 billion in 2048 (Rivlin and Wiener, 1988).

Projections could vary considerably from these numbers with small changes in disability assumptions and in the rate of cost inflation. For example, when disability assumptions are changed, the projected cost in 2018 ranges from $93 billion to $150 billion. Varying the inflation rate for long-term care moves the costs into a $66 billion to $245 billion range in 2018. Greater efficiency in delivering services — improved care planning, better targeting of needy populations, and more effective organization and use of volunteer services — also would affect cost estimates.

Declining birth rates imply that there will be relatively fewer workers available to help pay for long-term care when the elder population reaches its peak. Assuming birth rates stay low and no major change in immigration occurs, one may wonder if the general population will be able to carry the load or how best it might handle it. Much depends on such factors as the growth of the economy, the level of income relative to costs of living, the rate of increase in hospital and medical expenses, the sharing of long-term care costs between public and private sources, and the financial status of future elders.

Income and Assets

There is little doubt that over the past half century, the income and asset levels of the older population have improved. But the view that this population is now generally rich is not supported by statistics. Averages disguise the skewed distribution of wealth. Unfortunately, at a time of wide economic distress, the image of elders as "greedy geezers" who are exploiting the young becomes politically useful in attacks on programs like Social Security.

Elders with modest means hold much of their wealth in their homes. This asset is difficult to liquidate for short-term needs and carries overhead expense, taxes, or maintenance. Financial assets readily usable for short-term needs are unevenly spread across the older population. The median value of financial assets for elders in the top fifth as ranked by income was about $60,000, but it was only about $4,000 for the bottom fifth. The financial future for the next generation of elders may be brighter, depending on how well the United States prospers. Even then, prospects are unlikely to improve uniformly among older people or the general population.

While the very old will grow as a proportion of the expanding older population, they will have lower average income. Unlikely to be at work, their income sources — including private pension and social security — may keep pace with inflation but otherwise remain level. The oldest old, who depend heavily on social security and would benefit most from expansion of public programs directed at low-income individuals, will fare badly in times of retrenchment. By contrast, younger elders with more reliance on nongovernment sources (such as asset income and pensions) may be relatively better off as long as they escape catastrophic costs of health care.

The drain on elder incomes from health care, at a peak now, is projected to increase further and outpace their rising incomes. Low rates of private insurance among elders expose them to high out-of-pocket costs. The likelihood of incurring costs for acute and long-term care rises steadily with age, in reverse proportion to ability to pay.

Between now and 2011, because of the low birth rates of the Great Depression, the very old population will grow slowly. The years before 2011 appear to be an appropriate time in which to prepare to meet the needs of the baby boom.

3

Supporting Independence: The Role of Geriatrics

*We have to move away from the
episodic treatment-and-cure acute-care model.
This will require changes throughout the system,
from the curriculum in medical schools
to financial incentives to hospitals and others
who provide care for the chronically ill.*
—Paone, 1993, p. 32

Consider a man, aged ninety. He functions well, resides with his wife in an elevator building, and has no major health problems. Suddenly, he gets influenza and bacterial pneumonia. Arriving at a hospital emergency room with fever and cough, he is admitted to a traditional medical service, geared to middle-aged patients having single medical problems. After twelve days of treatment and bedrest, the patient goes home. The "system" has managed him reasonably well.

Now consider a ninety-year-old man also with flu and bacterial pneumonia. A widower living alone in a fourth-floor walkup apartment, he is found unconscious by his daughter and taken to the hospital. He is feverish, delirious, and dehydrated. Examination reveals he has experienced progressive memory loss and fits of screaming over the last six months and has long-standing diabetes and mild, inadequately controlled hypertension,

33

associated with occasional bouts of congestive heart failure. He also has glaucoma, vision loss, hearing loss, marked decline in general functioning for several months, weight loss of twenty pounds, malnutrition, urinary incontinence, major skin ulcers due to lying in bed for several weeks, and possible adverse reactions from the nine medications he takes.

Traditional medical services will control the flu, pneumonia, diabetes, and hypertension, but the other problems are beyond their resources. Cured of the flu and pneumonia, this patient will be discharged home but probably will be rehospitalized for worsening malnutrition and the other unresolved problems.

In a geriatrics unit, however, the staff of doctors, nurses, social workers, and other specialists understands the complications of geriatric illness and is not daunted by a screaming, frail old man who urinates in bed and tries to climb out.

The bedsores are treated by keeping him dry and changing his position in bed regularly. The incontinence is studied and found manageable by medication. The pneumonia is slowly cured. Aware that patients in the unfamiliar environment of a hospital often fall (producing hip fractures and bleeding in the brain) and that patients weaken when they have no exercise, the staff takes precautions in getting him up and moving about.

For his refractory behavior, special nursing and psychiatric care is given. A cognitive assessment determines he has early Alzheimer's disease. His vision and hearing losses are determined. A nutritional and rehabilitation program and a review of medications (to eliminate those unnecessary or harmful) are initiated in expectation of his discharge home.

Social workers, starting on the first hospital day, confer with his daughter and begin consideration of services to support him in his community or to gain admission to a nursing home. Care at home is found feasible with the daughter's cooperation and a plan of care involving periodic professional review.

Arriving home, the patient is attended for eight hours a day by a home health aide arranged through the social workers. Despite the Alzheimer's disease, he is able to remain in his apartment.

According to Howard Fillit, director of the sixteen-bed geriatric evaluation and treatment unit at Mount Sinai Hospital in New York, clinical research has shown that specialized units of this type, found in major medical centers, improve care of the frail elderly and save on costs of care, including those associated with rehospitalization.

The contrasting scenarios offered above begin this chapter's discussion of geriatrics. An understanding of this style of practice — adapted to the multiple needs of people with chronic illness or frailty — is central to the vision of health care reform offered in this book.

Geriatrics is the label given the special knowledge and skills applied through medicine, nursing, social work, and other professional disciplines for helping the elderly function, despite impairments, as independently as possible. Geriatrics is concerned principally with the following:

1. The patient's ability to function, to achieve the highest possible degree of independence
2. The patient as a whole person, including emotions, values, interests, and physical, mental, and social functioning
3. The patient's capacity for rehabilitation, new roles, and emotional growth (a key in all geriatrics planning)
4. Assisting the patient in compensating for limitations
5. Involving the patient and family in care planning
6. Adjusting physical and social environments to facilitate the patient's functioning
7. Using a team of professionals and paraprofessionals, as appropriate, to address the multiple needs of the patient and family

This comprehensive approach requires practitioners to have a thorough understanding of the patient. The doctor, nurse, and social worker can take little for granted or rely on stereotypes. Medical students are introduced to geriatrics with the dictum, "When you've seen one old person, you have seen one old person." The older population is far more heterogeneous than the younger adult population. As people grow older, treatments have

to become more individualized. A knowledge of what aging is—
and what it isn't—is crucial to effective care.

Diseases and Age

Diseases may appear differently in the old than in the young
adult and take different courses. An older person may not experience the chest pain of a heart attack. Infection may not be
accompanied by much of a fever. Behavioral problems may be
the expression of temporarily diminished blood flow to the brain.
To the uninitiated, these are oddities that confuse attempts at
diagnosis and treatment.

Complications also arise because very old patients tend
to have concurrent diseases and chronic conditions. For example, the drug of choice in dealing with an infection may adversely
affect the functioning of weak kidneys or adversely interact with
a cardiac drug. A treatment plan that works well for one patient will work poorly for another patient with a similar condition. The fledgling physician brought up on an understanding
of the prototypical "average forty-five-year-old, 154-pound male"
will have a lot of relearning to do to cope with increasing numbers of aged persons in the population.

The physician will come to understand that the encounters
of old people with the most powerful institutions and technologies of medicine have drawbacks, known as iatrogenic (practitioner caused) illnesses or losses. For example, the frail patient
is cured of pneumonia in the hospital, but the unrelieved bedrest
there undermines the patient's limited ability to walk.

Survival Mechanisms

Chronic diseases persist; they are rarely cured. They must be
lived with, and the wise physician knows how to help the patient
find a satisfactory way to live with the problem. Some patients
need little assistance besides medical care. They develop their
own strategies for survival by modifying their environments and
changing their self-expectations. Other patients need the help
of specialists as well as family members in coping with such

problems as loss of mobility, vision and hearing, and memory. The big secret of geriatrics is that most older people have surprising capacities to compensate for illness and disability. Besides having an innate ability to adjust to functional and social losses, they can be taught by others.

This ability to compensate contradicts the view that aging produces rigidity. People age differently, and aging is not unalloyed deterioration. Some people function well almost to the time of death. As science unravels the biology of later life, it is showing that diseases rather than normal aging processes produce weakness and incompetence. Laying aside disease, the restrictions appearing in later life reflect psychosocial and environment factors far more than genetics.

"To a large measure, the geriatric patient represents an organism with a restricted capacity to deal with a variety of stresses. Thus the geriatrician's role is to seek ways of reducing sources of stress and enhancing defenses. . . . What keeps all of us 'together' as we face life's assaults and challenges," observes Leslie S. Libow, a leader in geriatrics, "is a set of survival mechanisms. They keep the internal environment of the body in balance. Under such stresses as fever, fracture, surgery, and bereavement, an individual makes physiological and psychological compensations. So, too, the elderly person, but less easily and less effectively" (personal communication, April 1991).

Aging Is Malleable

The concept of aging as modifiable flies in the face of common belief, but it is scientifically demonstrable. The newer messages of gerontology are that people largely shape their own aging. Throughout their lives, people have the ability to promote their own health and contribute to society. Success depends on how they are equipped by nature (that is, by genetics), by self and family (motivation), and by society (access to education, decent pay and working conditions, medical care, and other institutions that promote healthful living).

The stereotype of increasing incompetence in old age feeds on a fragment of the biological, social, and psychological diversity exhibited by people in old age. Actually, most people do not lose competence over the long lifespan. They learn to adapt. They may fashion new roles and take up new vocations. While the diseased brain loses information, the normal brain is active across the lifespan, according to James E. Birren, a psychologist/ gerontologist. "Disease, more than age, plays the dramatic limiting role in the ability to function and make compensations," says physician/gerontologist Robert N. Butler. Older people gain in adaptive abilities at the very time that vulnerability to disease increases. An appreciation of this fact, central to geriatrics, can open the eyes of caregivers as well as patients to opportunities for improvement (Butler and Gleason, 1985, p. xvi).

Much can be done in old age to improve functional capacities: with cessation of cigarette smoking, lung function can become nearly normal for age; an exercise program can improve cardiovascular, pulmonary, and musculoskeletal performance; training and social interaction can keep people mentally sharp; drugs and psychotherapy can prevent depression due to bereavement from hardening into long-lasting behavioral problems (which may set the stage for further disability and acute illness). Thus, while reserve capacities are eroded by processes of aging, more of the remaining potential can be realized. Building up the aged body raises its odds of surviving an illness episode and achieving success in rehabilitation.

Conversely, counterproductive personal habits, social policies, and caregiving patterns (for example, poor diet and sedentary living, marginal roles for the retiree, scarce or unaffordable medical and social services, and unnecessary bed rest and inappropriate medication) can destroy functional capacity. Influenced by stereotypes, an individual may adopt dependent behaviors as natural for old age. George Burns, the nonagenarian comedian, noted that some people at age sixty-five begin rehearsing with a cane, and by age seventy they are a "hit."

Many people continue their lifelong productivity and others suddenly flower in late life, despite disabilities. The diversity of patterns confounds stereotypes of later life; they also condition the geriatrics practitioner to look for interferences in productive behavior, rather than to accept declining activity as unavoidable. Some older people act out stereotypes of old age and habituate themselves to disuse. The disuse syndrome can intensify cardiovascular vulnerability, obesity, musculoskeletal fragility, depression, and premature aging. The vernacular slogan—"use it or lose it"—states a principle of geriatrics.

In 1825, Benjamin Gompertz conducted actuarial studies that documented the fact that the chances of dying go up exponentially with age. The same is true of the chances of disability in performing ADLs, such as eating, dressing, bathing, and moving from bed to chair and back. Since Gompertz's time, average life expectancy at birth has improved enormously in industrialized countries, so that more of a birth cohort survives into old age. This is the period of highest mortality and morbidity rates, but recent analysis suggests that those who survive into the very oldest ages seem to live longer than Gompertz thought. Fragile as they may be, they seem to have an extra margin for survival.

Preventing Loss

Besides these biological patterns, geriatrics helps the patient contend with stereotypes and other prejudices that inhibit the capacity to make the most of life despite disabilities. An understanding of these influences allows the physician not only to expedite recovery and to maximize the recovery potential but also to prevent or cut short the course of functional losses.

The victories of geriatric medicine often evade the unpracticed eye. It is much easier to measure gains in acute care: An appendix becomes infected, it is removed, and life returns to normal. The patient who had been doubled up in pain is now back at work. The results of care are dramatic—a clear difference between life and death. The presumption is that the patient will recover previous functioning once the disease is cured. With geriatric care, what happens is that something does *not* happen to a person: less deterioration in an arthritic patient, or less abandonment of patient-preferred activities that make life worthwhile and allow self-reliance. "Burnout" of family members has been averted, and with it, the need to take up permanent residence in a nursing home.

The Whole Person

In geriatrics, an acute problem such as an infection often occurs as an overlay to one or more chronic diseases (for example, congestive heart failure and depression). One problem may
complicate treatment of another. Priorities in treatment must
be set according to personal importance to the patient as well
as medical urgency. The geriatrics practitioner may be able to
do nothing about hardened arteries but plenty to dissipate un-
due worries about survival, ability to work, and sexual capacity.

Because the patient with chronic conditions and frailty
is at constant risk of accident and slow or sudden deterioration
in health status, the physician-patient relationship should become a continuing process rather than consisting of episodic encounters. As Figure 3.1 shows, the care process ranges from
preconditions of a problem through acute care and rehabilitation to maintenance.

A Team Approach

Medical, social, and psychological knowledge must be accompanied by skills of communication, negotiation, and management. The key practitioner deals not only with the patient and
family members but also with other specialists in medicine, nursing, rehabilitation, and social work. Direct and indirect con-
tacts often are necessary with officials of public and private organizations that furnish money, authorizations for payment, and
services. For a heavily geriatric practice, this scope of activity
justifies a team effort.

Geriatrics often deals simultaneously with patient needs
on several levels: multiple medical, psychological, behavioral,
and social and environmental problems. The list of problems
will vary with time as issues are resolved, such as arthritic pain,
shortness of breath, poor hearing, hypertension, incontinence,
eating habits, safety hazards in the home, intrafamily conflicts,
loneliness, and mental depression. For the confused or demented
patient and family, counseling and referral to mutual help groups
and community services may be needed. The practitioner also

Figure 3.1. Extended Care Pathways.

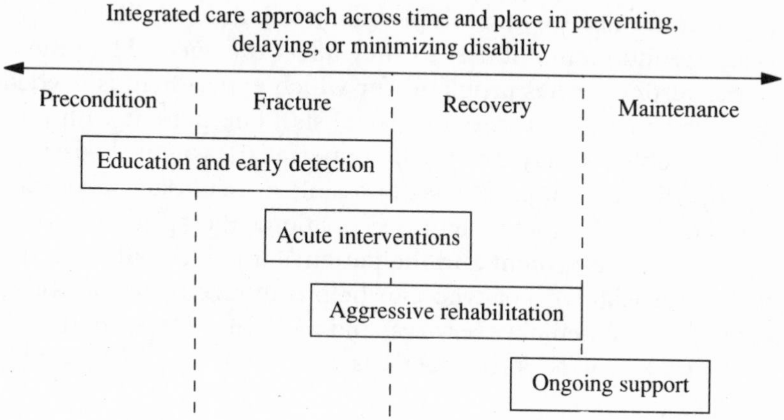

Integrated care approach across time and place in preventing, delaying, or minimizing disability

Source: National Chronic Care Consortium, 1993, p. 12. Used by permission.

has to be aware of financial and legal factors affecting behavior and health status, such as a near-poverty retirement income and marital conflicts.

Understanding the Patient's Wants

Success in preserving competence or minimizing losses depends on the ability of the practitioner to understand the patient as a whole person. Which problems does the patient say are most troublesome? What are the patient's priorities in treatment? How can interventions be least disturbing to and most facilitative of the activities prized by the patient? Sometimes, what is considered medically trivial may be enormously important to the patient: a small improvement in ability to walk, to hold the telephone, to retain urine for an extra thirty seconds. If the patient happens to be a caregiver to another person, the problems become more complex. At issue is preserving the symbiosis of a frail couple.

As frailty grows, the patient sees the doctor more often. The practitioner visits the patient who cannot come to the office.

Besides visits in the hospital, the practitioner sees the patient in the home and, especially, the nursing home. The geriatrics practitioner deals with such problems as balance (falls), incontinence, and mental illness as they affect the aged. The practitioner also identifies problems for which expert help is needed and then manages access to specialists. The patient with mobility problems may need a foot specialist, a neurologist, an orthopedist for gait problems of possible musculoskeletal origin, a geriatric nurse practitioner or occupational therapist to evaluate the home environment and the patient's use of a walker on the street, a social worker who can help organize transportation, meals, and homemaker services, and a pharmacologist to review drug intake for adverse reactions.

Maintaining Function

Preserving ability to function is a shared aim in geriatrics and rehabilitation. Besides helping the patient restore an ability, the specialist in rehabilitation seeks to prevent disability during treatment—for example, by taking steps to avoid contractures (tendon shrinkage) while a fractured wrist mends and to avoid bedsores for the individual confined to bed. In addition, disabled patients can be helped in adapting to their environment, which itself may be adjusted (for example, by removing obstacles to using the kitchen from a wheelchair). Expectations of the patients' adaptability need to be set realistically. According to T. E. Hunt (1978), ingrained professional attitudes that older people are not trainable may produce underachievement.

Mental health also is a major concern in geriatrics, since one in five elders has significant mental problems. Emotional problems may surface as physical disability develops. Behavioral changes may be the first clues to many physical problems: infectious disease, cerebrovascular problems, dementia, poor nutrition, a loss in hearing or vision, and/or a drug side effect. Behavioral changes also may indicate worry about finances, bereavement, and despondency over interpersonal conflicts.

Shadows in the Mind

Depression, a common disorder among elders, kills and maims in many ways. It can choke off attempts to obtain treatment, to recover self-reliance, and to maintain satisfaction with self and life. It may appear as lessened interest and pleasure in almost all activities, significant weight loss or gain when not dieting, too little or too much sleep nearly every day, feelings of worthlessness or excessive or inappropriate guilt, diminished ability to think, concentrate, and make decisions, and recurrent thoughts about death or suicide, possibly reflecting pessimism about old age in society at large.

Suicide rates tend to rise with age, particularly among whites. Elderly white men have the highest U.S. suicide rates, at 43.5 per 100,000 in 1989. This is about double the next highest white male rate (ages twenty to twenty-four). It is double or more the suicide rate for elderly black men. The white male suicide rate increases to 71.9 for the group aged eighty-five and older. For white women, the rate is 6.2 throughout old age. Statistics for black women were insufficient in 1989 to calculate rates. There has been a sharply increasing trend for white men after age seventy-four since 1970 (U.S. Bureau of the Census, 1992, p. 90).

Comprehensive Assessment

The care of old and frail patients should be approached systematically through a comprehensive geriatric assessment, which evaluates patients' ability to function in normal activities, their physical and mental status, their socioeconomic status, and their home, family, and other environmental circumstances. Social history, sexual history, and medication history — as well as a physical examination — are important in establishing a diagnosis, treatment goals, and the baseline condition of the patient, against which changes will be measured and interpreted. Assessments are done periodically to track the patient's status and to take timely precautions against further deterioration. Rather than cure disorders, which often is impossible, geriatric medicine focuses on improvement in functioning or in otherwise meeting the patient's need for an activity. A good example is the patient whose vision is worsening irretrievably but whose morale improves because special lenses and talking books become part of the treatment.

A geriatrics examination, including a careful history, takes more time than what is required for examination of younger adults. Loneliness, hearing impairment, mobility problems, poor memory and thinking, tendencies to underreport symptoms, and lack of clarity about problems and symptoms may lengthen the exam. All symptoms must be taken seriously because they may be atypical clues to a problem. Diseases may have different signs and symptoms from those in younger adults. Problems may be due to poor diet, ill-fitting dentures, the wrong prescriptions, taking medications in the wrong quantities (the body may metabolize drugs differently in old age), and the adverse effects of prescribed and over-the-counter drugs on memory, gait, and balance.

The nursing and social work assessments determine supports available to the patient and family in the community and at home, who the patient lives with, what medications the patient takes, how well the patient ambulates, whether the patient can feed himself or herself, the deficiencies in activities of daily living (ADLs), and availability of insurance and income to cover health care and other basic needs. The nurse determines what follow-up examinations may be needed to check on the patient's response to therapy.

These are some of the evaluations conducted by a team, usually including a physician, nurse, social worker, and other specialists as needed. The patient's own physician may make the referral to a medical center or other place for the comprehensive geriatrics assessment. Sometimes, the assessment is initiated when a patient or family member is unsatisfied or exasperated with uncoordinated diagnosis and care by various practitioners. It may occur as the result of a crisis in which admission to a hospital or a nursing home seems to be the solution, although the geriatrics-oriented practitioner well knows that institutionalization breeds dependency, induces confusion, and carries disease risks.

The comprehensive assessment may show treatable medical problems that permit options for care at home or in specialized apartment houses (with personal care services), supplemented by outpatient services, adult day care, and community volunteer programs. A plan of care is developed from the evaluation and discussion with the individual, family members or other informal caregivers, and the referring family doctor.

The plan has to involve the patient's regular physician, if willing, or a new physician who will provide primary care in solo office practice or as part of a group practice or health maintenance organization. No plan of care is adopted and put into effect without agreement between the professionals and the patient and principal informal caregivers. The processes of planning and implementation depend on trust and confidence.

Coordinating the health and social services in a complex plan is often beyond the capacity of family members. A care coordinator, also called a case manager, may be needed. This individual, often a nurse or social worker, negotiates for the patient with practitioners and with public and private agencies, which have their rules and limits. As we will see in the next chapter (on systems), the care coordinator plays a pivotal role in implementing the original plan and its revisions as conditions change.

A Social Assessment

In line with the objective of supporting the patient's self-reliance and life-style is the geriatrician's questioning about the patient's needs for help in preparing meals, shopping, housecleaning, getting into or out of bed, dressing, and bathing. How much assistance is needed, when, and who provides it? How often does the patient leave the house? Does the patient have transportation and a telephone? With whom does the patient live, if not alone? Does the patient have a confidant? In an emergency unrelated to health care, whom does the patient call? What are the patient's income level and income sources, and is income sufficient for food, shelter, housing, drugs, heating, and transportation? Is the patient receiving social services, and what are they?

What did the patient eat yesterday? (Kane and others, 1980, pp. 323–355).

Family Dimension

The physician discovers if there are family members and identifies those who have influence with the patient and can help in an emergency or for long periods of time. The socioeconomic inquiries may show whether the patient has enough money for an adequate diet, transportation, and a properly heated apartment and whether the neighborhood is considered safe.

Since family members furnish the greatest part of long-term care, their capabilities are important to the professional team serving the at-home patient. Family members can be trained to take care of many care problems themselves or jointly with visiting nurses, therapists, and home aides. Even complex cases can often be handled more appropriately and economically at home than in the hospital (Rossman, 1978). But when family members are over-stressed and physically incapacitated, the patient's health and safety may be jeopardized to the point where hospitalization or a stay in the nursing home is needed.

Environmental Assessment

Environmental assessment is done by questionnaire and by visit (by a nurse or social worker). It covers housing, need to climb stairs, safety of neighborhood, and safety provisions in the bathroom. A home visit should provide information on cleanliness of living quarters, obvious hazards, signs of neglect (such as old food in the refrigerator or unwashed dishes), sufficient food on hand, and evidence of alcohol abuse.

The assessments are completed and discussed by the appropriate professionals. A set of problems and treatments have been identified. With a diagnosis in hand, the professionals formulate a prognosis, or statement of what may be expected of the patient under the proposed or prescribed regimen of care. This statement is crucial. A well-informed, realistic prognosis can prepare a patient and family members for encouraging or discouraging transitions. Nonetheless, prognostication remains more of an art than a science: responses of patients to interventions are highly varied, and setbacks as well as unexpected recoveries often occur.

Receptivity to the prognosis is influenced by the doctor-patient relationship. If the relationship is marked by candor, affection, and respect, the issue of relocation to a nursing home can be raised with a minimum of fear and resistance. It need not represent the threat of loss of control over the patient's life.

Ageism and False Labels

The labeling of patients as "senile," "demented," and "incontinent" is another danger. Labeling and stereotyping of patients are obstacles to realistic treatment; opportunities for proper evaluation, for rehabilitation, and for restoration to normal life may be missed.

As gerontologist Robert N. Butler puts it, the elderly patient runs the risk of getting "the senile write off," which trivializes the complaints of the elderly. It is not uncommon to hear that the complaint is an inevitable outcome of old age, which is not treatable, or for caregivers to deny that the patient has a problem when the problem is most likely terminal.

Pessimism in patient as well as practitioner is fed by a general social phenomenon: discrimination against the elderly, or ageism. (The term *ageism* originated in the 1960s and gained currency through the work of Butler, 1975.) This prejudice can have disastrous clinical consequences in the form of therapeutic nihilism. It feeds on the notion that aging itself is a disease — inevitable and irremediable.

Historically, ageism owes much to the industrial revolution and scientific medicine: industrialists saw the older worker as worn out and inefficient; early scientific medicine saw only the elderly sick and characterized aging accordingly. Old age, poverty, and disease were thought to be a common and synergistic triad. Poverty bred disease, and disease bred poverty. Age prejudice was self-confirming by deterring care and research.

Geriatrics was generated as a response to ageism in the early twentieth century; Ignatz Nascher, an American physician who saw lives wasted by therapeutic nihilism, coined the term *geriatrics* and wrote one of the first texts on the subject (Butler, 1975).

Advocacy for the patient is needed today to overcome ageism. Coordination, or case management, is necessary because ready-made systems of geriatrics are lacking or inadequate. Systems have to be assembled, in many instances across professional, administrative, and programmatic boundaries — not only are health and social services in different sites involved, but third-party payers (government and private), housing, transportation, and legal services are also part of the picture. Often, the geriatrics-oriented physician has to begin the process.

The geriatrics-oriented physician works with the patient in various locales in providing continuity of care. The patterns in health care system use explain why acute care and long-term care must be considered together (Densen, 1991).

Producing Able Personnel

Professional educational and service strategies are needed for widespread implementation of the practices just described. Despite the fact that one-third of all patient expenditures in the United States is for older people, geriatrics is only starting to be taught in medical and other professional schools.

Proposals for improving access and quality of long-term care all require many more geriatrics-oriented practitioners. Only a tiny fraction of health care professionals have any proficiency in geriatrics. Shortages of physicians, nurses, allied health staff, long-term care administrators, and other personnel exist.

Professional training appears only loosely synchronized with the growth of the elder population. One reason is that geriatrics runs counter to the heavy focus of many medical schools on specialty and subspecialty training of physicians (Kane and others, 1980). The knowledge and skills needed for effective coordination of services in various sites of care, from home to institution, have little place in conventional medical education (Pfeiffer, 1977).

After World War II, as private insurance took hold, most American doctors became specialists rather than generalists. Health insurance reinforces medical specialism and its technologies rather than primary care by general physicians, pediatricians, and geriatricians. Insurers prefer to pay for procedures rather than time spent with the patient.

Attempts to reinvigorate primary care have reached into payment arrangements. The Physician Payments Review Commission, set up by Congress to make recommendations on paying for doctor services under Medicare, concluded that some procedures are overcompensated for on the basis of resources used. Geriatrics is not well paid by Medicare. Per unit of time, Medicare places a much higher value on the performance of physicians' specialty procedures than on their "evaluation and management services" in primary practice (for example, history taking, physical examination, diagnosis, and care supervision). For a lengthy visit (one hour) or for a procedure requiring ten minutes, Medicare may pay the same $101. While the commission recommended changes favoring primary care geriatrics, the improvements appeared to be modest. The research for the revisions touched only lightly on geriatrics problems.

Geriatrician Shortage

The shortage of physicians skilled in geriatric medicine was studied by the Rand Corporation in 1980 (Kane and others, 1980). It offered a range of estimates of potential needs for "geriatricians" in 1990 to serve in primary care, in consulting practice, and in academic life. Another set of estimates concerned the need for "geropsychiatrists," since one in five elders has significant psychiatric symptoms. The Rand study represented an attempt to bring medical care into line with demographics.

The estimates considered the effects of delegating some physician activities to nurse practitioners and physician assistants, but these practitioners are themselves in short supply.

For 1990, assuming no change in per patient allocation of time resources, Rand estimated that 8,300 to 13,400 geriatricians would be needed. They would act chiefly as consultants to primary care doctors. Some would take academic posts.

If more time were allotted for elder patients, the range would
be 10,000 to 16,700. The numbers could be roughly halved if,
instead of serving all elders, the focus was on persons seventy-
five and older. The study also noted increased needs for physician assistants, geriatric nurse practitioners, and other health
care personnel.

That was the view from 1980. The study's authors concluded that their estimated geriatrician levels for 1990 could not
be achieved in ten years. They were correct. In 1986, the National Institute on Aging found: (1) only 100 physicians entering
practice in geriatric medicine and geriatric psychiatry each year;
(2) 242 available fellowship positions in geriatrics medicine; (3)
only 4 percent of medical students taking electives in geriatrics;
(4) geriatrics courses rarely required by medical schools; and
(5) few residents in internal medicine and family practice taking
geriatrics training (National Institute on Aging, 1987). However,
a major step was subsequently taken when the American Board
of Internal Medicine and the American Board of Family Medicine developed a certificate of proficiency in geriatric medicine.

Medical education has responded slowly for several reasons: professional prejudice against geriatrics as an incursion
in internal medicine and other specialties; Medicare payments
to physicians for primary care, as the Physician Payments Review Commission noted, are disadvantaged compared to payments for surgery, radiology, and subspecialties; weak financial
support of new training programs by the federal and state governments; the strained finances of medical schools; and a shortage of career positions in geriatrics.

Today's personnel in geriatric medicine is no more than
one-tenth of the lower Rand estimates. Using the Rand meth-
odology, the National Institute on Aging estimated the need for
geriatricians in the year 2000 at double the 1990 Rand figures.
To achieve this would require a formidable shift in medical training. More realistic is a strategy that would involve continuing
education, or short courses for professionals already in practice.

It is not clear whether the United States is likely to have a
glut of physicians in the future. Even if so, the serious shortage
of physicians trained in geriatrics probably will worsen (Figures
3.2 to 3.4). The government could stimulate geriatrics through

Figure 3.2. The Growing Gap: Current/Expected Number of Geriatrics-Trained Doctors Versus Projected Need.

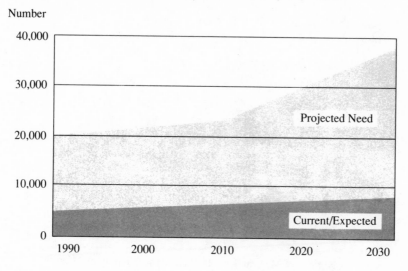

Source: DelPonte, 1992, p. 8. Used by permission.

Figure 3.3. Gap in Geriatrics Medical Faculty: Current Versus Recommended Faculty by the Year 2000.

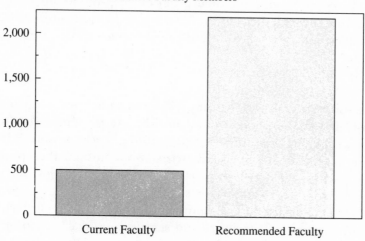

Source: DelPonte, 1992, p. 20. Used by permission.

Figure 3.4. Medical School Curriculum, 1988–1989:
Medical Schools Requiring Geriatric Coursework.

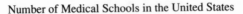

Number of Medical Schools in the United States

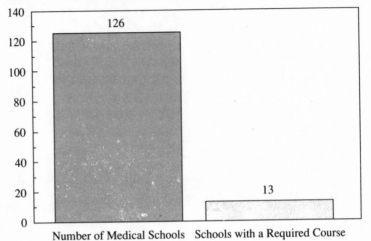

Number of Medical Schools   Schools with a Required Course

Source: DelPonte, 1992, p. 17. Used by permission.

grants or low-cost loans to offset the heavy costs of medical education, through changes in payment for physician services in
geriatrics, through a national program to promote long-term
care, and through the training of care coordinators, nurse practitioners, and other health and social service professionals.

A Variety of Therapists

The estimates of shortages of geriatrics-trained physicians are
paralleled for dental and other health care personnel serving
elders (National Institute on Aging, 1987). These personnel include dental hygienists, podiatrists, occupational therapists,
physical therapists, social workers, home health aides, nurse
aides, chore aides, audiologists, psychologists, and dietitians.
To this list must be added administrative personnel to deal with
the management of facilities and services and teachers to prepare the practitioners and support personnel. On the basis of
population increases and more care per patient, the number of

registered nurses (RNs) estimated for 2000 is 2.33 to 2.96 million, about double the 1984 level. This assumes more RNs in nursing homes, because the number of residents will increase. As the age and disability level of residents increases, the professional time per resident per day will rise. Instead of twelve to seventeen minutes (the 1980s pattern), about one hour of RN time will be needed. Total nursing time in 2000 will be 3.5 hours per resident per day, one-third provided by RNs, one-sixth by licensed practical nurses (LPNs), and one-half by nurse aides (National Institute on Aging, 1987, pp. 56–67).

Nurses in Geriatrics

Estimates of the need for nurses for community care and home care programs depend on as-yet undetermined specifications for the organization and financing of service delivery. The extent of involvement of informal caregivers also makes a difference in numbers of paid professionals needed. Assembling a stable and adequate pool of semiprofessional personnel—such as aides for nursing homes and home care programs—will require major changes. Career paths will have to be defined, pay and benefits improved, and training provided to ensure the quality and effectiveness of service. In most categories, training programs exist, but the overall effort probably fits the label of "token." Training support by government has been trimmed to fit current fiscal pressures, leaving the future to take care of itself.

The Labor Department estimated in 1987 that there would be 9.8 million jobs in health services in 2000, up from 6.5 million in 1986 and 3.4 million in 1972 (U.S. Bureau of the Census, 1987). The larger growth rates will be in nursing and personal care facilities and in outpatient care and other health services. According to the Labor Department study, the growth of the over-eighty-five population in particular will produce job opportunities and health care expenditures.

Modernizing the U.S. health care system to deal effectively with the issues of an older population will require bold steps to change the goals of professional education and the supporting financial arrangements. Meanwhile, the systems for delivering services—the organizations whose methods of delivering services require new kinds of personnel—must be reoriented, too.

4

Putting Long-Term Care Together: Systems at Work

In essence, a nonsystem currently exists,
within which the chronically ill and aged
are easily lost and frequently ignored.
—Joint American Medical Association/American Nurses Association
Task Force to Address the Improvement of Health Care
of the Aged Chronically Ill, 1983, p. 1

Geriatrics-oriented systems are mixtures of institutions, agencies, practitioners, aides, family members, and volunteers. A system can take many different forms, but at the core is a triad of functions: assessment, care planning, and care coordination. This triad is necessary to overcome fragmentation in the balkanized world of acute and long-term care services.

The traffic in this world for an elderly population was traced in a pioneering study by the U.S. Agency for Health Care Policy and Research (Densen, 1991). The diagram in Figure 4.1 is based on data involving physicians, hospitals, and nursing homes. For home health programs, data are available concerning entry from hospitals but not from the community. Other data gaps exist. The diagram indicates nothing about personal care at home, adult day-care centers, hospice programs, and many other key services. Figure 4.1 does make the important

54

Figure 4.1. Annual Movement of Persons Sixty-Five and Over Through the Health Care System.

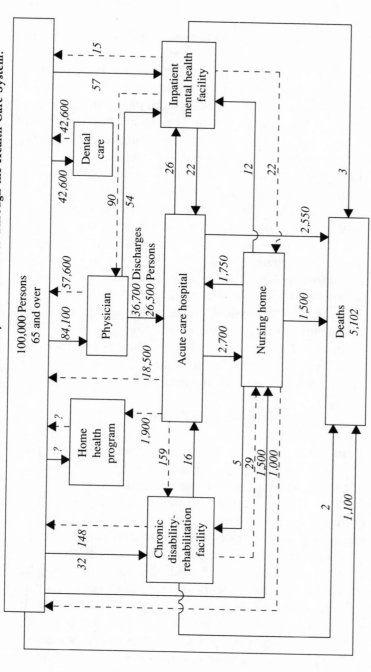

Note: ———➤ =Movement to more restrictive/intensive care setting.

- - - - ➤ =Movement to less restrictive/intensive care setting.

Source: Adapted from Densen, 1991.

point, however, that acute and long-term care facilities exchange patients. The hospital is the major pathway to nursing home care. About 10 percent of hospitalized elders are discharged to nursing homes for skilled or intermediate care. As a result of a change in Medicare payment of hospitals, the posthospital use of nursing homes increased. About 24 percent of all elders admitted to a nursing home return to the community. Reentry from the nursing home to the hospital is frequent.

The organized community care program appears more and more important to the quality of late life. Fragmentary information indicates that 33 percent of elders use community services. Some 8 percent of all elders use home care, with 11 percent of the old-old using home care in a year. Other parts of the system are rehabilitation facilities and inpatient mental health facilities. To provide continuity of care, the geriatrics-oriented physician works with the patient in these locales.

The mosaic of individual practitioners, service groups, and volunteer and family participants is tied together by the care coordinator. This professional person brings together the health, social service, and other information needed to carry out a plan of care for the patient and family.

Individualizing Services

The goals of the system are to promote the frail or disabled patient's self-reliance to the greatest extent possible and to enable a quality of life satisfying to the patient and family.

A well-run system serves the individual in the *least restrictive* environment (such as the home instead of the nursing home). "Infantilizing" the patient through excessive servicing is destructive to patient and family. The system has to be flexible and inventive to deal with a variety of needs. By using the strengths of the individual, family, neighbors, and volunteer organizations, the system economizes on paid services. A course between over- and underservicing requires staffs to be expert in evaluating needs and strengths and, with patient and family participation, in creating and carrying out a plan of care and adjusting it as circumstances change over time.

An effective plan of care incorporates a division of labor between paid and unpaid caregivers. Relieved of burdens better handled by trained workers, families continue to give emotional and basic care. Contrary to myth, families are unlikely to withdraw from the scene when professionally directed home care services are begun. The astute nursing home likewise will encourage family members to play the kind of caring role that only they can carry out.

Reliable assessment/planning tools already exist for the operational needs of a benefits program. They are being applied in prototype systems to measure the kinds and intensity of deficiencies in ADLs, instrumental activities of daily living (IDLs), and mental status. When personnel who do the ratings are well trained, their findings are accurate, replicable, and usable by various service providers and administrators. The information is useful for monitoring the cost, quality, and appropriateness of what the delivery system does.

Kinds of Systems

Among the varieties of systems is the ready-made system, such as a social and health maintenance organization, or SHMO. There is a single administration for medical, nursing, social, and supportive services. The SHMO, described later, provides acute care as well as long-term care.

At the other extreme is the ad hoc system assembled by a care coordinator chosen by the patient and family. The coordinator may be an independent operator or part of an agency. Often a licensed social worker or nurse, the coordinator works with practitioners and other service providers already chosen by the patient, such as the family physician. The coordinator also links the patient and family with other services they need. The coordinator may spot and remedy inconsistencies and gaps in the service fabric and may ensure good communication among the providers and family. Actually, few chronically ill or disabled patients and their families will need all the resources of the full system. But most patients will need some at one time or another.

Instead of confronting and wandering among agencies and complex administrative processes, the patient and family deal with a single planning, administration, and accounting point. When in a ready-made or ad hoc arrangement, the coordinator serves as an interpreter and an advocate for the patient. In a ready-made system, the coordinator also may have a responsibility for minimizing costs to the program. A conflict of interest can arise between what is best for the patient and the program's rules on expenditures or cost controls. A truly professional system explains its rules clearly before enrollment. The coordinator has a duty to make any conflict explicit and find a solution by obtaining an exception to the rules or by helping to secure services outside the program.

Chapter Three described the goals of care. The current chapter focuses on the structures of an operating system to achieve those goals. The basic functions include making an assessment and care plan to integrate various professional and nonprofessional services (medical and nonmedical, paid and volunteer), ensuring the quality of care, and managing the costs of services.

Example of Care at Home

Chapter Three, in explaining the geriatrics approach to a patient having both an acute care problem (pneumonia) and other problems, discussed a minisystem called the geriatrics evaluation and treatment unit of a medical center. For the patient in that scenario, who belonged to no system at the outset, a post-hospital system was being fabricated through discharge planning and referral to home care and outpatient services. What if a patient lives in a community that has a geriatrics-oriented system already in operation?

Consider the case of a ninety-three-year-old former accountant, Mr. Abel, who was a member of a ready-made system. Bacterial pneumonia sent him to the hospital for two weeks. By the time the infection cleared, the hospital staff and his physician had worked out a simple discharge plan in consultation with Mrs. Abel. At eighty-three, she functioned well enough despite arthritis to help her frail husband with his problems, including bowel and prostate cancers, and to maintain their household.

On Mr. Abel's return home, visiting nurses came to give him convalescent care for two weeks. A long-term care team — a social worker and RN — had been in touch with the doctor and hospital to prepare a long-term care plan. The plan was discussed with the Abels and a son, who was available by phone. The plan helped the family organize itself (for example, by scheduling short visits and dividing bill paying and other duties), make use of community services (such as a meals-on-wheels program), and know when to ask for professional assistance.

Mrs. Abel was the only daily caregiver; their children were not available and neighbors helped only occasionally. The main issue in their plan of care was to support Mrs. Abel in her caregiver role. If *her* health and vigor gave out, *he* would need much more service at home, and the couple might have to leave their house for congregate care housing. Or Mr. Abel would need a nursing home.

Difficult times were in store for Mrs. Abel because of his cancer and because of his vulnerability to falls and accidents due to poor hearing and cognitive problems, infection, and other major stress. Under the plan of care, a homemaker came twice a week for three hours to do heavy cleaning and give Mrs. Abel a chance to leave the house for shopping or other activities. The homemaker was trained to report changes in health and functioning. The team scheduled itself to see the Abels every month and made occasional contact with their doctors. Finally, by facilitating the use of community services for transportation to clinics and meals-on-wheels, the team added yet another set of supporters and observers.

Mr. Abel was in stable condition for two months. Then he worsened. He died six months after returning home, just as the family was considering nursing home placement. Mrs. Abel decided to remain in her household. A plan of care was developed with her participation and the cooperation of her physician, son, and neighbors. The plan included periodic visits to the physician, daily phone calls by friends, monthly calls by the care coordinator, and assistance with household maintenance by neighbors, members of her church, and volunteer chore workers from a senior citizen center.

Because they had joined the long-term care system and paid their premiums of $35 per month each, the Abels were protected for home care expenses up to $6,000 a year each, a limit that was not exceeded under their care plan. They might easily have spent twice or triple this amount if they had not had the care coordination, for which there was no charge by the system. Had the Abels not belonged to the system, they would have had to pay for each practitioner visit for maintenance or long-term care. (The posthospitalization home health care was part of convalescence paid for by Medicare.)

Through care coordination, they were spared overspending and excessive servicing that might have depleted their savings. Medicaid was out of the question for the Abels. Their savings and pension income disqualified them. Applying for Medicaid would have been an act of desperation for middle-class people like them. Besides, their state Medicaid program had an inadequate home care benefit.

The Abels were served by a delivery system that met geriatrics objectives of timely, family-oriented support, assessment and care planning, preventive care, continuum of care, and monitoring/review. They were assisted but not "infantilized." Mr. Abel lived his remaining months in the environment he preferred without welfare stigma or fear of impoverishment from the costs of needed services.

Tokenism in the United States

Few Americans have the advantages of a comprehensive long-term care system. Most existing systems are small, provisional, and incompletely tested. Promoted under government rather than private insurance auspices, these few comprehensive long-term care systems show that fragmentation in financing and services can be overcome.

Many industrialized nations have policies for providing medical, social, and personal-care services that help middle-class people live at home. Swiss and Germans buy the personal care.

Financial status of close family members is considered when determining whether an elder is eligible for a public subsidy. In France, social security pays at a fixed rate for the medical component of care in residential facilities, and the residents pay for room and board or apply for welfare assistance (Tilly and Stucki, 1991).

Israel provides home care for people with severe impairments who can live in the community and offers cash benefits to the family if needed public services are unaccessible. Japan recently started a program with home care and day care. Australia provides home help, personal care, home nursing, and respite care to persons at risk of institutionalization. Nursing home residents must contribute 87.5 percent of the amount of the country's basic pension payment.

Some countries use assessments to determine the need for institutionalization. Australia has regional teams to evaluate disability levels; the Netherlands has a national assessment system for home care; Israel has a team of nurse, social worker, and eligibility worker. In Japan, welfare and health departments plan service delivery to elders, with care coordination to unify providers of long-term care.

More than any other industrialized country, the United States leaves it to the middle-class elder and family to carry the financial load and assemble a care program. Paid home care is erratically covered by public and private insurance. The chief paying organization is neither an insurance program nor a public health program but a welfare program — Medicaid — and it does not pay until the individual is impoverished.

For the middle-class individual and family, the choices are hardly encouraging: do without, buy what you can for as long as you can, then enter a nursing home on public charity. The United States is distinguished by weak, incomplete, and poorly funded networks of home care and community-based services. Most elders pay privately or do without.

Relatively little is done to produce housing programs integrated with supportive services, especially social services and personal assistance. In congregate housing, services for residents are added as they become frail and disabled. Some nursing homes, responding to Medicare, have become less like a domicile and more like a hospital. Originally, they were boarding homes with nursing. This kind of service is furnished on a spectrum that includes the intermediate care facility (less "medicalized" nursing home) on one end to foster homes and board-and-care homes on the other. Appropriate placement is crucial.

Important to geriatrics are two major aspects of system making: linkage of acute and long-term care (symbolized by the cooperation of the hospital, nursing home, home care agency, and other service providers), and the integration of medical and nonmedical services (symbolized by doctor and social services).

The needs of a patient vary over the duration of a chronic impairment: occasionally, an acute illness takes priority, but the presence of chronic conditions often complicates and prolongs the treatment. This presents a complication not only for the clinician and family but also for the mix of institutions and funders involved in services. Although Medicare does not cover long-term care, Medicare is influenced by it. For example, the geriatrics unit at Mount Sinai Hospital in New York reported that 40 percent of admitted patients had major nutritional deficits. A maintenance matter — poor nutrition or erratic drug taking or cleanliness — may send the patient to the hospital with an acute illness. The benefits of more effective custodial or maintenance care accrue to Medicare's providers and financiers. Given the marginal incomes of many elders, the flow of patients between acute and custodial care is also a flow of jurisdiction between Medicare and Medicaid. This gives one program an interest in the other. Patients in Medicaid nursing homes get doctor care largely paid for by Medicare.

Hospital Economies: Unsystematic Reforms

Hospitals have problems with the dichotomy between acute and custodial care. They take financial losses when frail patients have completed a course of acute care but are not ready to leave. Medicare pays hospitals a lump sum based on the patient's assignment to one of about 400 diagnostic-related groups (DRGs). The payment is the same regardless of the duration of the patient's hospital stay and use of services. If more rather than fewer items of service are provided, the hospital may lose money; the reverse is also true. The hospital hopes to cover its service costs and retain funds for teaching, charity care, and capital expansion.

In some hands, the DRG method — a reaction to previous "blank check" payment arrangements — may undermine patient care. Although convincing evidence is lacking, some fear that the DRG method may encourage inadequate treatment in the hospital and premature transfer to home. The DRG payment covers no more of the spectrum of care than the hospital portion.

The hospital may find itself caught between the payment incentives to discharge patients and good reasons to keep them, such as no bedspace in a nursing home or lack of informal supports at home. The costs for this portion of a hospital stay may be wholly denied or only partially recognized for payment by third parties like Medicare.

About 5 to 7 percent of Medicare patient-days have been attributed to patients in transition to long-term care. The patient is paid for as receiving an "alternative level of care" (ALC); the payment rate is lower than for acute care. Under Medicare's prospective payment system using DRGs, the hospital sees the ALC patient as a fiscal loss. The loss occurs because the payments are less than cost and because the hospital cannot fill the beds with patients for whom higher payments would be received.

The DRG arrangement should have been accompanied by an expansion of home care and nursing home services. The lack of systematic approaches tends to complicate problems for the fragmented U.S. "system." Examples are available from the cost containment efforts in Medicaid and Medicare. Some states have made an effort to restrain Medicaid spending by imposing moratoriums on nursing home construction in the last decade, with repercussions for hospitals as well as the elderly. Meanwhile, Medicare restricted the use of home health benefits and adopted a lump-sum payment to hospitals by DRGs. At the same time that policymakers spoke encouragingly of home care, the policies made it difficult to discharge Medicare patients to home care or to nursing home care and forced hospitals to absorb the costs of hospitalization extended by the nonhospital restrictions.

In the mid 1980s, the United Hospital fund in New York reported, fewer elders were receiving care at home. "Policymakers continue to tout home care while seeking to constrain its growth and control its costs," the Fund said. "The victims of this fragmented and at times inconsistent policy process will be the elderly who need, but cannot afford, care" (Fox, 1989, p. 2).

Selected Prototypes

In the following paragraphs, we look at several types of health care systems.

Private Organizations

The systems described below are veritable islands in a sea of fragmentation. All together, they probably serve fewer than 100,000 persons.

Social and Health Maintenance Organization (SHMO). This is a variant of the health maintenance organization (HMO), in which physician and hospital services are under unified administration and financing. The SHMO, conceived by gerontologists in the early 1970s at Brandeis University, adds long-term care services to the HMO spectrum. The SHMO offers organized and cost-controlled services financed mainly by Medicare and a long-term care premium.

Four SHMOs with 16,000 participants, who are Medicare or Medicare/Medicaid beneficiaries, are being tried out in a federally approved demonstration program. The four SHMOs are in Brooklyn, New York, sponsored by a nursing home; in Minneapolis, Minnesota, sponsored by a housing enterprise; in Long Beach, California, sponsored by a community agency; and in Portland, Oregon, sponsored by an established HMO.

For each enrollee, Medicare pays the SHMO an amount equal to the average annual expense of Medicare beneficiaries in the locality. This amount, or capitation, is for the standard

Medicare services plus additional benefits (such as preventive medicine and outpatient drugs) made possible by SHMO efficiencies. Long-term care is covered by a supplementary "premium" paid by each SHMO participant.

The SHMO participant agrees to receive all covered services from the SHMO. Only in the event of emergency or pre-authorization will the SHMO pay for services delivered by other practitioners or organizations. The participant cannot shop around and expect the SHMO to pay for services. This limitation is the crux of "managed care." All services are prescribed and coordinated by a single management (Leutz and others, 1990).

If expenses exceed income from Medicare, Medicaid, and the supplementary premium, the SHMO pays the difference out of its own capital. Any surplus or profit may be shared by staff (such as through higher pay or bonuses) and clients (through lower cost sharing or more benefits). Maintenance of quality of service is a key issue in applying cost controls.

For long-term care in 1990, SHMO members paid premiums ranging from $25 to $57 per month (in the range of Medigap policies but much less than private long-term care insurance policies). Medicaid members of the SHMO pay no premium for the long-term care. The premium supports a limited amount of long-term care in the nursing home and at home ($6,000 a year in one plan, $12,000 in another). Care coordination is available at all times, even after the dollar limits are exceeded (but the beneficiary pays the cost of the "excess" long-term care).

The fear that long-term care benefits cannot be controlled is baseless, according to a group evaluating the SHMO demonstration project (Leutz and others, 1990). Moreover, beneficiaries sometimes refuse paid services to which they are entitled. The SHMOs have found that many patients and family members would rather meet most, it not all, custodial care needs (such as bathing) on their own. As expected, the SHMO data reveal that paid or formal services are used at a relatively high level by people who live alone, the most disabled and least ambulatory, and the most socially isolated. Most SHMO long-term care is home care. Nursing home admissions are chiefly for rehabilitation and respite care (Walter Leutz, Bigel Institute, Brandeis University, personal communication, April 1992).

The SHMOs have had problems in getting started. Regarding them as a Trojan horse for Medicare expansion, the Reagan administration delayed their funding for several years (until 1985), costing them a marketing advantage over many private insurance policies. Because the public mistakenly believed that Medicare and supplementary private insurance (Medigap) covered long-term care, the SHMOs had to educate potential customers about their unique benefits package. They had to teach the value of integrated acute and long-term care services while trying to sell policies.

Partly to keep premiums competitive with Medigap insurance, SHMOs have had to guard against acquiring too many elders with greater-than-average service needs. Three of the four SHMOs employ a quota system to obtain a financially safe mix of patients. Between 5 and 9 percent of SHMO members were certifiable for nursing home admission under state standards (Leutz and others, 1990). Long-term care benefits have therefore been limited, but the limits are rarely exceeded.

After four operating years, the four SHMOs cleared a break-even point on total operations (despite high marketing and enrollment costs). At the seven-year point, they appeared to have demonstrated their viability and readiness for inclusion in Medicare on a regular basis. The possibilities of private insurance based on coordinated long-term care are being explored.

The expansion of HMOs into SHMOs would seem to be an attractive possibility and much easier to accomplish than building SHMOs without a preexisting HMO base. Competition with long-term care *indemnity* insurance, a cheaper product focusing on nursing home care and depending on physician judgment, will be a problem. It may complicate any attempted expansion of the SHMO concept in the marketplace. The SHMOs may have their greatest effect in showing HMOs that expansion into long-term care is feasible.

A Housing-Based System. An example of a private organization specializing in preserving community living for the most frail

elderly is On Lok in San Francisco's Chinatown. Based in a congregate housing project, On Lok provides adult day health care
for severely impaired clients. A tribute to its effectiveness is that
only one in twenty of its clients is in a nursing home on any
single day—a much lower number than expected for these people, who are certified eligible for skilled care in a nursing facility. Hospital use also is surprisingly low for this population.

Directly or by contract, On Lok provides social, nursing, rehabilitative, and medical/hospital services, recreational
activities, meals, personal care, and transportation to and from
home for its 300 clients, who have an average age of eighty-one
and are mainly poor. Medicare and Medicaid pay for benefits
at a negotiated per person rate. The rates represent savings of
11 percent for Medicare and 5 percent for Medicaid. Non-
Medicaid participants pay a monthly premium for some benefits. The savings are attributed to lower hospital use and to
all-inclusive rates On Lok negotiates with hospitals, doctors, and
other providers.

The On Lok model may be applicable to developmen-
tally disabled children, hospice patients, and individuals with
AIDS. Like frail elders, AIDS patients may have multiple medical and psychosocial needs requiring coordinated, comprehensive services. The model, like other systems of long-term care,
could be integrated with private insurance, Medicare HMOs,
and congregate housing.

National Chronic Care Consortium (NCCC). This group of fourteen organizations of hospitals and multi-institutional systems
bridges acute and long-term care services. These systems are
developing geriatric care networks for the chronic care of older
adults. A key element of a network is a comprehensive hospital
system and a comprehensive long-term care network. They may
be under the same auspices or may be allied in serving a common clientele. The network provides managed care for heavy-
use, chronic care clients, particularly with a capitated approach
covering acute and long-term care.

One NCCC member is the Group Health Cooperative
of Puget Sound, Washington. This is an HMO with two hospitals and an inpatient unit in a community hospital, a Medicare-

certified home health agency, a hospice agency, and a skilled
nursing facility. There are twenty-five primary care and four
specialty care centers, an outpatient geriatric assessment clinic,
a network of home and community volunteer services, and a
primary care team of geriatric nurse practitioners and physicians. The team services 750 cooperative members who are nursing facility residents.

Huntington Memorial Hospital in Pasadena, California,
provides acute and community-based long-term care, a Senior
Care Network. The hospital is part of an initiative by the Robert
Wood Johnson Life Care at Home program. This has resulted
in a long-term care insurance product under joint sponsorship
with a national insurance carrier. The hospital has a federal grant
to improve in-home care and is a site for a Medicaid waiver
program providing alternatives to nursing home placement. A
geriatric assessment center was set up in 1993.

The Philadelphia Geriatric Center is one of the outstand-
ing long-term care organizations in the country, particularly
for applied research in geriatrics and geropsychiatry. The center
is one of the first long-term care providers to become hospital
certified. Its special care unit for Alzheimer's disease was a
pacesetter. Offered are a complete range of institutional and
community-based long-term care programs, senior housing, and
acute care (nonsurgical). Care coordination has a long history
at the center. The center's partner is Philadelphia's Albert Ein-
stein Medical Center, which has 600 hospital beds, extensive
outpatient services, a 102-bed skilled nursing and rehabilitation facility plus other geriatric services, a geropsychiatry program, a hospice service, and a program providing health education, health promotion, insurance counseling, and medical
claims assistance to 35,000 older persons.

Rochester General Hospital and Park Ridge Health Systems are developing geriatric care networks in Rochester, New
York. The hospital offers comprehensive services to the frail
elderly with care coordination (the On Lok model) using capitation financing through Medicare and Medicaid and other
arrangements. These arrangements are to include long-term care
insurance (like the model of the New York plan discussed in

Chapter Six). The network links up with senior housing (apartments at below-market rates built by private and public capital) and a Community Coalition for Long-Term Care. Park Ridge Health Systems includes an organization for chronic care with a continuum of services and a senior housing retirement village.

Continuing Care Retirement Community (CCRC). In its most comprehensive form, this system offers housing, health care services, and long-term care in its own or affiliated nursing home or through a staff of visiting nurses and aides. The CCRC participant pays a sizable entrance fee and monthly payments for the housing and services. This option is primarily for the relatively rich.

Federal-State Programs

Spurred by fast-rising costs of care in nursing homes, the federal-state Medicaid program expanded into home and community-based care in the 1980s. Ordinarily, if a state desires to add this care, it must be available statewide. The state may ask for a waiver of this requirement in order to experiment with expansions for particular areas or groups. A waiver (known as a *2176 waiver* for the section of the Social Security Act that authorizes it) carries a proviso that the experiment will not add to federal fiscal support for the state Medicaid program. Federal aid to states is also available through the Older Americans Act, which helps to support a network of state offices on aging and area agencies on aging. The "aging network" conducts federally aided, nonwelfare programs, such as senior citizen centers, meals-on-wheels, volunteer services, transportation, legal aid, housing, employment, and ombuds services.

In long-term care, the area agencies on aging (AAAs) provide information and referral services to older persons, whether they are officially classified as poor or not. In some states, the program may also provide for some in-home care. While the Older Americans Act provides for coordinating community-based health and social services, the act confers no authority over the primary government programs that provide health care (Medicare and Medicaid) or over social services funded through federal block grants. However, a state may take the initiative of consolidating services for which it receives federal grants under Medicaid and the Older Americans Act.

Oregon Program. Using a Medicaid waiver and the aging network, Oregon exemplifies state-based systems that unify the community and institutional aspects of long-term care. However, the Oregon program does not integrate acute care and long-term care.

The responsible state agency for Medicaid and non-Medicaid long-term care is the Senior Services Division of the state department of human resources. The non-Medicaid program is Oregon's Project Independence, supported by the Older Americans Act and state funds.

Oregon's objective is to minimize nursing home placement. State officials say that the use of foster homes (small homes directed by trained and licensed proprietors) has been a major factor in achieving savings over traditional service patterns and has improved the quality of life and care for elders. Charges that the state went too far — that many patients in group homes should be in nursing homes — were dismissed by a federal study.

Oregon relies heavily on care managers for assessment of clients and the arrangement of services. Eligibility of individuals for public services is based on financial status and need for service. The care managers assist those who do not qualify for publicly funded services in finding other aid. The coordinators prepare plans of care, including nonmedical services, and arrange placements and other benefits (such as food stamps). Cases are monitored or reviewed by the coordinators, who are nurses and social workers. They screen patients who are, or soon will be, eligible for Medicaid, to determine the best placement for them. They also help nursing home residents make transitions back to the community. Other functions include helping communities to organize volunteer services and to investigate complaints of abuse.

The National Governors Association acclaimed the Oregon

experience, noting its control over long-term care costs at a time when other states were swimming in deficits from nursing home expenses. But some observers believe that Oregon's experience may not be easily repeated elsewhere, because of its politics, culture, and rural character.

Programs in Other States. Massachusetts combines various funding streams to support nonprofit home care corporations in twenty-seven service areas. The corporations — often AAAs — subcontract to local provider agencies for care coordination, homemaker services, personal care, home-delivered meals, transportation, adult social day care, and chore services. Respite, companion, laundry, protective, and emergency shelter services are provided as well. The corporations hire nurses to help in hospital discharge planning. One corporation assigns representatives to hospital emergency rooms to make community care arrangements, thereby avoiding some hospital admissions.

The Massachusetts program serves 6 percent of all elders in the state, mostly people who live alone and have incomes under the federal poverty level. State officials believe the home care program has paid for itself in savings on nursing home admissions.

Other states besides Oregon and Massachusetts serve as laboratories for systematizing long-term care. Preadmission screening has been applied to candidates for nursing home and community care in several states. In *New York,* people found to be disabled enough for institutional care may be offered a program of enriched home care. *Texas* finds this approach to be cost-ineffective, seeking instead to identify people *before* their need for care reaches the nursing home level. *Wisconsin's* approach to long-term care seeks ways of protecting older caregivers from burnout and illness, since they are providers of long-term care for others. Respite care and adult day care are available, and Wisconsin pays individuals for performing coordinating tasks for themselves or others.

New York has the Expanded In-Home Services for the Elderly Program (EISEP). This non-Medicaid program brings care coordination, homemaking, and other services to about 5,000 persons — chiefly women over seventy-five — who live alone and have an income no higher than 150 percent of the poverty level. The few clients above the 150 percent level share in the costs of care. EISEP clients generally are impaired in six of nine IADLs, or needs for help with shopping, transportation, housework, and meal preparation. They also have impairments in one or more ADLs. Some 40 percent have no family member or other informal caregiver. On entry into the program, 40 percent of clients surveyed in 1989 required therapeutic diets, 12 percent had gone without eating at least one day a week, and 24 percent had to take five or more medications a day.

Care coordination and assessment services are without charge, but clients pay for home services on a sliding scale according to income. Most clients get homemaker and personal care (averaging almost ten hours a week) or housekeeper/chore services (averaging almost four hours a week). Because the assessment is based on a protocol used by Medicaid and other New York State agencies, it need not be repeated if a client shifts programs.

EISEP is funded entirely by state and local governments. The program has demonstrated an enormous unmet need; it has also shown that the services can be furnished relatively inexpensively. With thousands on a waiting list, the program is caught between state fiscal problems and a growing middle class demand. The waiting list for assessment or services is long, due to lack of funds and a shortage of in-home workers. The population needing or eligible for EISEP services was estimated at 100,000 in 1989, or twenty times the monthly number being served. Local programs had to limit or eliminate outreach (discovery) efforts.

Home Care as a Public Health Service

Bordering Minnesota and North Dakota, the Canadian province of *Manitoba* offers a wholly public model of universal entitlement to comprehensive health care. It provides comprehensive long-term care for people of all ages without regard to income or earmarked contributions. The system appears fiscally controlled, socially responsive, and popular.

In Canada, each province participates in national health insurance by meeting federal standards, but each has its distinctive mix of services, administration, and financing. The Manitoba program insures coverage in hospitals, day hospitals, nursing homes, and physician offices. Insurance also covers prescribed drugs. There is no private health insurance under Canadian law for services covered by public insurance.

Home care is not an insured program but a service of the Manitoba health department, which receives federal aid on a different basis from insured services. This makes no practical difference to providing a continuum of acute and long-term care.

The problems of coordination and impoverishment encountered in U.S. long-term care are, literally, foreign to Manitobans. The long-term care program has no reason to investigate anyone's income and asset status or require a "spend down." The case example involving the Abel family earlier in this chapter can be considered a depiction of a Manitoba program if references to financing are ignored.

Because long-term care is considered family care, both the patient and the family member providing care can be served as a unit. Patients receive long-term care on their own request or on referral by family members, physicians, hospital discharge offices, and other sources. A district health department office is responsible for patients living in the district.

The district office offers assessment/care planning and home care at no expense to the patient. The assessment process engages the patient's own physician. The first decision concerns what level of care is needed. The site of care is determined by medical, nursing, and psychosocial factors, including patient and family preference.

A plan of care is generated from a nursing–social work evaluation of patient and family situation. The assessment and care plan documents are prepared so that they can be used by all providers of health and social services; the document eliminates duplication of effort and expedites action.

In the hands of an implementation team that knows the community, the plan makes the most of volunteer and other community services. By emphasizing self-reliance, the plan is frugal. It builds on, rather than supplants, patient and family strengths and uses volunteers, aides, and practitioners with the minimum necessary skills.

When nursing home placement has to be considered, a special panel of geriatrician, nurse, and social worker is convened to hear the reasons why. The process ensures that all factors have been considered. The patient may be asked to see a geriatrician or specialist for additional medical evaluation. If a recommendation for the placement is approved, the patient will be put on a waiting list for the nursing home of choice or placed elsewhere until the preferred institution has an opening. Alternatively, the patient could be kept at home with nursing and other home care services.

To help families maintain patients at home, the system provides adult day care and respite services whereby patients are placed temporarily in a nursing home so other family members may have a vacation. Special attention is given to fragile individuals who may need preventive services (including adaptation of their homes with safety devices and minor structural renovation), placement in congregate housing, and volunteer services (transportation, meals-on-wheels, friendly visiting).

The system is not without its problems—specifically, large caseloads and insufficient involvement of the primary care physicians (Kane and Kane, 1987, p. 313). Progress is being made in obtaining closer physician cooperation, and administrators have developed guidelines on caseload volume: more than 100 cases per nurse or social worker, or 200 per team, make the tasks of evaluating and monitoring difficult and expensive. Mostly, a stressed team tends to err on the side of too much service. The system's home care component drastically reduces the need for institutional care.

At any one time, nearly 13,500 persons are in the program, which serves 16.5 percent of the elderly population. The versatility of home care is seen in the care-level equivalent of persons admitted to home care in 1990–91: about half would have been in hospitals, and just over one-third would have been in nursing homes. Most home care patients improve to the point of being able to manage themselves or to manage with some help of family and friends.

Despite a growing elderly population, Manitoba has escaped a rapidly growing institutional population. If there were no such home care program, the province would have had to pay for hospital and nursing home expansion. The cost of home care (including administration and care coordination) in 1990–91 was $216 per month. This compares with $2,204 a month for nursing home care (Fineman, 1992).

Most nursing homes in Manitoba are nonprofit facilities. They are paid on the basis of a budget. The few for-profit homes are paid on a formula related to the nonprofit homes' budgets. The number of facilities is small enough so that every one of them is familiar to government officials and professionals. The tone of provincial regulation appears less adversarial than government regulation in the United States, officials comment. The basic stance is one of helping the institutions do their job. Abuses of patients and payment arrangements seem to be rare.

Does the provision of government benefits for long-term care prompt families to desert elderly patients? According to Betty Havens, the health department gerontologist, in testimony before the House Select Committee on Aging in July 1985, the answer was clearly no. "I consider home care as the most enabling of programs to insure that families can and will continue to care for older family members. Universality of home care and insured nursing-home care are further guarantees of support by families, not deterrents. [Some] 80 percent of the care provided to persons over the age of 65 is still provided by the family and/or members of the informal support system. This rate was 80 percent before home care was introduced and 80 percent before the insured nursing-home program was introduced. It is still 80 percent."

More examples of systems of long-term care in different degrees of integration with acute care could be provided. The key point is that enough has been shown to move the United States beyond tokenism.

5

Holes in the Safety Net:
Medicaid, Medicare,
and Medigap

*Attempts to reformulate
the system of geriatric care delivery
without appropriate reorganization of
the general health-service system
are doomed to failure.*
—Maddox and Manton, 1989, p. 71

The previous chapters have highlighted the conditions and needs of the older population, the ideals and practices of geriatrics (not widely known or available), and the few systems that coordinate or unite a variety of health and social services to help maintain or achieve as much independence as possible for the population at risk. This chapter and the following one concentrate on the payment arrangements that require reform in order to achieve effective care of the elderly and others at risk of chronic disability.

Where the Money Goes

Today's fragmented and confusing mosaic of services cannot be replaced without reforming the underpinnings of a similarly disorganized set of financing arrangements. Each financing element

76

moves under its own rules, with contrary and overlapping effects, eligibility requirements, benefits packages, and methods and levels of payment. From the standpoint of the previous chapters, the programs delivering and financing long-term care are antisystems, bedeviling and obstructing patients and families, practitioners, and administrators.

The Three M's and Long-Term Care

The chief payment sources for older people with long-term care and associated needs are — in this order — themselves and their families, Medicaid, Medicare, and Medigap. Each source has its own dynamics. The government programs are in financial spasm due to deficits at the federal and state levels. That any experimentation has occurred in Medicare and Medicaid toward the goals of systematized long-term care may be counted as miraculous. Patches of these programs may represent workable forerunners of such systems, given the right financing approaches. In Chapter Six, we discuss private long-term care insurance, as yet a tiny contributor whose potential to support geriatrics and long-term care systems for most people is doubtful.

Painfully clear from our perspective is that improvement of the health and functioning of the older population is secondary to financial gamesmanship among the programs, the "musical chairs" of shifting costs elsewhere, and the "blindman's buff" of complex and shifting eligibility rules.

Nonsupport of Comprehensive Geriatrics

None of the major American health insurers — commercial insurance, Blue Cross and Blue Shield, or Medicare — supports comprehensive geriatrics and systematized long-term care broadly and coherently. At best, they are reluctant supporters of home and community care services. The very services needed by the frail and disabled are beyond the mainstream financing patterns that evolved primarily for working adults.

It is left to a public assistance program, Medicaid, to evolve — largely in desperation about nursing home costs to state governments — community-based long-term care systems. Medicare, the main health insurance for elders, is not the main payer of long-term care. That is Medicaid.

Principally because of outpatient drug and long-term care exclusions, Medicare pays only for 40 to 45 percent of elders' health care expenses on average. This is a lower percentage than when the program started in 1966. This kind of performance turns elders to Medigap, private supplementary insurance.

Because of third-party payers' shortcomings, there is no American safety net against impoverishment from expenses of chronic illness and disability. A systematic bias against Americans with long-term care needs exists:

1. Medicaid sacrifices precious opportunities to preserve individuals' ability to function by waiting until they lose financial independence.
2. Medicare omits long-term care and services to prevent or mitigate chronic disability.
3. Medigap policies (private insurance supplementing Medicare) close no long-term care gaps.

An examination of these programs shows us impediments and paths to long-term care security.

Medicaid: The Partial Safety Net

A program for poor people, Medicaid may support the full slate of geriatrics and long-term care services (Figure 5.1). Preventive medical care and outpatient drugs, for example, may be covered along with rehabilitation, homemaking services, and social services. Medicaid pays for custodial care in nursing homes in all states. But it pays for custodial care at home only in some states — chiefly in New York, followed by California, Pennsylvania, and Michigan.

The benefits slate is not uniform across the country. The eligibility rules vary, too. A patient eligible in one state may be ineligible in another. Payment levels also vary, but in general, states are low or erratic payers for those physician services not

Figure 5.1. Where the Medicaid Dollar for the Elderly Goes, 1989.

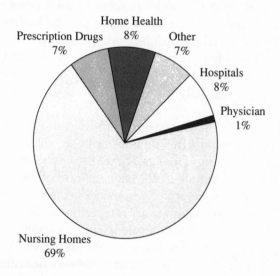

Source: Reilly, Clauser, and Baugh, 1990.

covered by Medicare. In sum, Medicaid is not a monolithic national program with uniform benefits, eligibility standards, and payment rules, as is Medicare.

Someone once said that a program for poor people is likely to be a poor program. One might add that, despite its potential, Medicaid is a poor environment for geriatrics.

A Variety of Programs

Medicaid is the generic term for fifty different state programs plus those in the District of Columbia, Puerto Rico, and U.S. territories. With federal aid, these programs help pay for the health care of poor people in certain categories (for example, old persons, blind persons, disabled persons, and families with dependent children). But Medicaid does not cover all the categorical poor. Only one-third of elders defined as poor are covered by Medicaid. Some decline to apply for benefits, either because they are ashamed or fear being put away in nursing homes.

The state programs must meet federal requirements in order to receive from 50 to 80 percent of their costs from the federal government. The poorer states get the higher percentages of federal matching funds. State programs must provide a basic set of benefits, including hospital, doctor, and nursing home services. Home care is optional. Medicaid spends over $20 billion a year, chiefly for nursing home care, for about 2.8 million elders.

Medicaid is the fastest-growing item in state operating budgets, with expenditures increasing faster than the general inflation rate. Nursing home and other expenses, chiefly for the elderly, absorb about half of all Medicaid funds. The fiscal problems have required some states to consider tax increases and have led to restricting the number of nursing home beds. Even so, the rising numbers of frail and poor elders suggest that problems will persist and worsen if no solutions are found. While some states have been reluctant to expand home care benefits, the nation's governors see home care as a definite part of a solution.

Waivers for Long-Term Care

In Chapter Four, we mentioned the optional program for states known as the 2176 waiver program (it takes its name, as noted, from the authorizing section of the federal Medicaid law). This program supports home and community-based services for limited populations. The waivers are based on the premise that savings will be realized by treating patients in the community rather than in nursing homes; however, this premise is questionable. A community care benefit may attract new patients in greater numbers than are diverted from nursing homes.

An exclusionary tactic, fending off more spending, is the use of unrealistic income-and-asset thresholds for receiving benefits. In a few states, the qualifying income level is the federal definition of poverty. In 1990, this was $6,268 for the elder living alone ($121 a week) and $7,905 for a couple ($152 a week). Most states use a *lower* income threshold. Applicants may be disqualified if they have too much in assets—below $5,000 in most states, not counting burial fund, home, and automobile.

In some states, Medicaid benefits may be available to persons who are "medically needy." That is, while income exceeds the state standard, the figure for income less medical expenses may place the individual below the standard. The assets test may be met once assets are used up, a process called a *spend down*.

Gateway to Care: Indigence

The indigence rules used to apply the income and assets of a couple to the spouse in a nursing home. This often left the community-living spouse unable to pay rent and other necessities. Recent federal rules enable the community-living spouse, at state discretion, to keep up to $18,000 a year ($230 per month) and $70,000 in assets. However, if the ill spouse remains at home, the regular Medicaid income and assets limits apply.

The extent to which nursing home expenses "convert" private-pay patients to Medicaid is not clear. Many persons are believed to convert within a few months. Others are said to convert to Medicaid before entering because resources were depleted by expenses of home care, prescribed drugs, and previous nursing home stays (Rice, 1989).

The incidence of spend down grows as length of stay in a nursing home grows. Some 36 percent of stays are covered by Medicaid from the beginning. The conversion from private-pay status to Medicaid status — a definition of spend down in the nursing home — may occur for individuals living alone in 4.5 percent of admissions in thirteen weeks, and in 22 percent of admissions after six months to a year. The corresponding figures for couples were 6 and 15–18 percent. Nursing home expenses are by far the largest out-of-pocket (that is, uninsured) burden among health care services. Of the 1.3 million elders who had at least $3,000 in out-of-pocket expenditures in 1985, nursing home expenses comprised 82.5 percent of the out-of-pocket spending.

The statement that Medicaid has become a middle-class nursing home program is often heard. Some state officials complain that people who are not poor have found lawful ways to qualify for Medicaid by giving assets to children or by placing assets in certain kinds of trusts. If the gifts or trusts occur thirty months or more before applying for Medicaid, no nursing home coverage is withheld. Within the thirty months, however, Medicaid may refuse to make payments in whole or part. The situation is different for Medicaid home care applicants; under federal law, there is no "look back."

Despite suspicion of the practice of "paper" spend downs, there is scant documentation. The countable (nonhouse) assets of most elders are relatively low, and so there is usually little for spending down. States may place liens on houses when single elders become permanent nursing home residents or after they die.

The eligibility process of state Medicaid programs tends to delay help until crises have become financially and medically hard to manage. By then, many elders have lost the chance to keep some independence and community life. These results are antithetical to geriatrics.

Several provisions to improve Medicaid were salvaged from the repealed 1988 Medicare Catastrophic Coverage Act: states were required to buy into Medicare for all elderly and disabled Medicaid recipients so they would be freed of user charges. States could receive federal matching for covering the marginal poor (up to 150 percent of the federal poverty level) and for liberalizing the provisions applying to community-living spouses of nursing home residents. The easing of Medicaid restrictions could reduce the market for private indemnity coverage.

Medicare: Not a Geriatrics Program

Medicare was modeled after job-based private insurance: heavy protection for short-term hospitalization and medical specialists, light for primary care, and no preventive medicine. Geriatrics was not part of the design. (See Figure 5.2.) Political and fiscal safety were thought to lie within the familiar bounds of private insurance, with some exceptions. Medicare did expand on private insurance by incorporating a short-term home health benefit and an "extended care" or posthospital convalescent benefit delivered in skilled nursing facilities. These are in Medicare (Part A), which wage earners pay for through payroll taxes.

Figure 5.2. Where the Medicare Dollar for the Elderly Goes, 1987.

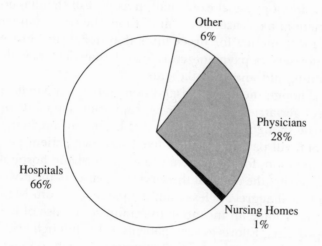

Note: Total exceeds 100 percent due to rounding.
Source: Waldo, Sonnefeld, McKusick, and Arnett, 1989.

The Acute Care Nursing Home

The program's use of nursing homes and home health care confuses people, who tend to associate these services with long-term care. The Medicare law contains a specific prohibition against paying for custodial care in any setting. What Medicare pays for in a nursing home is basically rehabilitation care. It pays for home health care only if certain conditions are met: a physician needs to prepare a plan of care for a patient who is essentially confined to home. The plan must involve an RN or other skilled practitioner (such as a physical or speech therapist, as authorized by a physician). A homemaker or home health aide may be involved incidentally.

Medicare (Part B) covers most physician services. Routine medical checkups are excluded. Only recently have Pap smears, mammography, and flu vaccination been added to the few preventive services. The preeminent Medicare method of paying doctors is according to procedures done for the patient. Payment is made for a visit, including the taking of the patient's history and a physical examination as part of the diagnosis or treatment of a disease. Per unit of time, the physician tends to make more money for procedures than for visits. Procedural or fee-for-service payment tends to underpay doctors with time-consuming old and frail patients.

Though the above observations show that Medicare underpays geriatrics, the Medicare capitation payment method might be thought to encourage this branch of medicine. The program will pay an HMO a fixed sum per patient per year, or a capitation, for the patient's total medical and hospital care. HMOs accept the risk that the service expenses of their Medicare patients will aggregate less than the payments from Medicare. Thus, they have an incentive to minimize the use of hospitals and specialists. Efforts to keep patients well—through health promotion and disease prevention measures—seem to make sense from financial and geriatrics viewpoints. Theoretically, an HMO could apply any savings to support a non-Medicare benefit, such as an amount of long-term care.

However, profit making may conflict with ideals of serving patients. HMO financing arrangements do not preclude stratagems to avoid enrolling old and frail persons. The Medicare program has dropped or criticized a few HMOs for curtailing necessary services or failing to pay for them. Perhaps no financial incentive guarantees quality of care and fairness of coverage in the absence of a professional dedication to ideals of service.

Custodial Care Issues

The U.S. Health Care Financing Administration supervises the Medicare program and its paying agents—Blue Cross and Blue Shield and private commercial insurance companies. The boundary that insurance draws between acute and custodial care is irrelevant to the clinical objectives of geriatrics: helping the patient reach as high a level of independence and quality of life as conditions allow. Medicare may reject bills on grounds that hospital, nursing home, or home health agency care was not medically necessary to improve or maintain the patient's condition. But this approach overlooks the many instances when, if deprived of relatively inexpensive custodial care, the patient will indeed need a doctor or hospital for an acute illness.

The vague boundaries between types of care produce tensions and dilemmas for geriatrics-oriented physicians. Recognizing that the Medicare patient cannot afford needed short-term maintenance care at home or in the nursing home, the physician may have to devise ways of writing progress notes that will qualify the patient in the eyes of the paymasters. On the other hand, under pressure to economize on each case, the paymasters try to read between the lines for disqualifications. Meanwhile, Medicare's hospital payment policy creates pressure on physicians to discharge a patient as early as medically justified. But sometimes it makes sense to retain a patient in the hospital even though medically ready to leave. For example, there may be nobody at home to supervise or help the weak patient with meals, cleanliness, and taking medications. Or the home is an unsafe environment because of barriers, hazards, and abusive family members. An unappealing substandard Medicare payment is available to hospitals for an "alternate level of care" while the patient waits for home care and other arrangements to be made. The Medicare hospital payments policy would make better sense if there were a long-term care program in the community ready to pick up where the hospital leaves off.

Medicare Payments for Geriatrics

A survey of six experts in geriatrics and fifty office-based clinicians indicated that Medicare's benefit structure and payment arrangements fail to support high-quality office care in geriatrics (Muller, Fahs, and Schechter, 1989). Nor are house calls reasonably paid for. The responding clinicians typically made house calls and nursing home visits, and they did so far more frequently than physicians in general despite the payment level.

The mean fee for a standard first visit at the time was $70, and half the surveyed clinicians said this fee did not cover costs. The average time they spent with older patients was thirty-eight minutes, far less than the hour or more recommended by the six experts. Only one-fifth of clinicians spent an hour or more with an elderly patient on the first visit (the experts' preference), and under half spent more time with patients over eighty than with younger elders. In some countries, fees rise with age of patient; not so in the United States.

Underpayment for primary care for frail and disabled patients strikes geriatricians as pennywise and pound foolish. Most of the clinicians in the study said the benefit structure limited their diagnostic and treatment options. Many said Medicare ignored preventive procedures and failed to cover certain activities (for example, foot care, home care) adequately. Most said Medicare did not cover the nonphysician services needed to complete a comprehensive diagnosis or a plan of care. As for incentives under capitation plans, one expert asserted that HMOs required physicians to process a high number of patients per hour, rewarding them for doing fewer procedures—a pattern of practice he characterized as poor care. Another expert felt HMOs would mature and become more age sensitive.

Not surprisingly, the surveyed physicians called for expanded physician services, higher payment for office visits (based on time spent with the patient), and compensation for preventive services. The gaps they identified in the survey are filled through SHMOs via capitation payment, as discussed in Chapter Four.

Medigap: Toeing the Line

Medicare covers only 45 percent of all beneficiary health care expenses. Aware of this, two-thirds of Medicare beneficiaries purchase private supplementary insurance, called *Medigap policies,* for protection against financial catastrophe. This may take the form of hospital and doctor charges that Medicare does not pay. A basic Medigap policy may cost upward of $600 a year. These policies rarely cover long-term care, outpatient drugs, or any other services not covered by Medicare.

The door to supplementation was left open when Medicare was designed with deductibles and coinsurances under advice from private insurers. These cost-sharing devices, supposed to help deter frivolous use of hospitals and doctors, are hardships in a low-income population like the very old. Since physicians and hospital administrators are the gatekeepers to hospitalization, one might argue that deductibles make more sense if directed at them rather than at patients.

Sales abuses, other exploitations of the elderly, and confusing provisions convinced Congress after many years to structure the Medigap market. Among the reported frequent sales abuses was the misrepresentation of some Medigap policies as covering long-term care. Agents have sold some older people several Medigap policies, even though only one will pay under coordination-of-benefits clauses. Such tactics have destroyed the financial security of some elders.

Insurers now may offer a basic plan and nine possible expansions. No plan may duplicate Medicare benefits. All plans must cover the 20 percent coinsurance on doctor services and certain hospital charges: the coinsurance incurred after the sixtieth day, the 90 lifetime reserve days, and 365 days in addition. At higher premiums than for the basic plan, the expansions may cover the Part A deductible ($684 in 1993), days 21–100 in a skilled nursing facility ($85.50 per day), the Part B deductible ($100), a proportion of fees for outpatient prescribed drugs up to a maximum, preventive medical services, and short-term at-home help with ADLs during recovery from an illness, injury, or surgery.

Medigap insurers must pay out benefits averaging at least 60 percent of the individual premium and 75 percent of the group policy premium. The policies do not have to cover preexisting illnesses for six months after purchase.

The annual premium ranges from $400 to $1,600 a year. An estimated $16 billion is spent annually on Medigap policies. For the most part, these policies do little for geriatrics and long-term care, and their premiums are often hardships for low-income elders. Sales commissions, advertising, and administrative expenses are part of the maximum 40 percent overhead allowed for Medigap policies. This compares with 3 to 5 percent overhead for Medicare, which, of course, has no sales costs.

According to testimony by *Consumer Reports* staff before the House Ways and Means Committee, the pre-reform Medigap market wasted $3 billion annually because of duplicative health insurance policies and low benefits payoffs. It noted that some state insurance departments had weak enforcement procedures and that abuses could be expected to continue. Consumer Union representatives urged Congress to prevent the emerging market for long-term care insurance from following the Medigap market's behavior.

The financing arrangements briefly surveyed in this chapter are part of a system that is seriously out of synchronization with the needs of a population with chronic disabilities. The American health care system resembles the physician who prescribes inappropriately or counterproductively for the patient; the system and the doctor may be hazardous to someone's health.

Medicaid, Medicare, and Medigap miss important elements of a sound prescription. In the next chapter, we examine private long-term care insurance to see if it has any of the missing ingredients.

6

Private Insurance and the Illusion of Protection

You can expect to pay premiums for many years before you subject any claims for long-term care. During this time, you are trusting that the company will pay the claim.
— Polniaszek, 1992, p. 3

Private insurance for long-term care is so recent that it probably should be considered experimental. In 1980, fewer than 100,000 policies were in force. By 1991, an estimated 2 million had been sold. Premiums were about $1 billion a year. The impact of these policies remained relatively tiny in 1992: they paid for about 1 percent of nursing home care. Perhaps one in twenty-five elders had the insurance.

The earlier policies followed the acute care insurance model, focusing on institutional coverage determined by medical necessity. Home care was covered lightly. Later policies introduced refinements at higher premium rates. They replaced medical necessity with functional and cognitive assessments as the catalyst for benefits.

In contrast to the service-benefit approach in hospital insurance, long-term care insurance offers a cash indemnity per day in the nursing home. Home care is covered at a per diem rate that is half that for the nursing home. This flat-rate approach makes it difficult to tailor home care to the diverse and changing needs of individuals.

Premiums vary by options: a higher premium buys a higher per diem, a longer period of coverage (such as six years versus three years), a shorter waiting period before benefits start (for example, thirty instead of ninety days), and an inflation adjustment. A nonforfeiture provision — allowing, in the event of a lapse or cancellation, refund of some premium payments and interest, or the equivalent in paid-up coverage — would also raise the price of a policy.

Initial premiums are higher for older purchasers (though the rate does not go up because the policyholder ages) and for individuals who have higher likelihood of needing long-term care. These risk factors may be health as well as social factors — such as living alone.

In the early 1990s, the annual premium for a relatively comprehensive policy was in the range of $1,500–$2,000 for a sixty-five-year-old person and double for a seventy-nine-year-old. Couples pay a multiple of these amounts. According to United Seniors Health Cooperative of Washington, D.C., nearly all insurers price their policies to return no more than about 60 percent of revenues. Thus, 40 cents on the premium dollar is reserved for profits and costs of sales, marketing, and administration. The Cooperative says that companies oppose higher payouts in benefits, even to 65 percent, on grounds that the insurance would not be profitable enough for the risk.

Sales abuses have been reviewed by six Congressional hearings since 1987. Companies pay agents between 40 and 90 percent of first-year premiums — potentially a strong incentive for high-pressure sales tactics. According to the General Accounting Office, an estimated four out of ten policies are sold to people with insufficient incomes and assets. Companies surveyed by the General Accounting Office (1992) expected that an average of six in ten policyholders would let their policies lapse in the first ten years. The reasons were not clear, since the figures may include "free looks" and exchanges, as well as inability to pay.

Another problem arises from lapses in conjunction with the level premium structure. Under this structure, a large portion of the premium in the early years is for prefunding the expenses expected in the later years. This prefunded amount of money is lost to the policyholder when the policy lapses.

Expected forfeitures are used in setting prices. This helps to keep rates lower than otherwise would be the case. Under pressure of consumer groups and state insurance officials, newer policies include nonforfeiture provisions. But the premiums are higher, and this makes it harder for agents to sell the insurance and for policyholders to retain it.

Consumer and Insurer Questions

Because of the interval between sale and use, called the "long tail," today's policies mainly are untested. An insurer may collect premiums from a policyholder for more than a decade before being called on to pay benefits. Insurers lack precise data for determining how much profit or loss may be generated by a new policyholder or group of policyholders in the future. In the interim, the insurer may invest the premiums and collect interest on these funds. If it turns out that the benefit payouts exceed income and reserves, the insurer could declare bankruptcy, raise premiums, or sell out.

The uncertainties of long-term financial stability and profitability are scant comfort to prospective buyers and insurer stockholders. An insurer can set a premium that appears most likely to cover a worst-case scenario, or underprice a policy to attract customers, reserving the right to raise the price later.

Inflation Protection

An Achilles' heel of the policies is "inflation protection." Typically, this feature raises the indemnity level and the premium by 5 percent per year, even though nursing home costs historically have risen much more. Chances are low that an insurance policy bought at age fifty or sixty will be used before age seventy-five. In the interval, costs of living will go up, the costs of care will rise more rapidly, and individual or household discretionary income is likely to decline. Health care expenses rise as a proportion of the average retiree's budget. Premiums for Part B of Medicare and for Medigap policies will increase. Costs of outpatient drugs also can be expected to rise. With advancing age, it becomes harder for the individual to cover the premiums. In the fifteen- or twenty-year interval between starting the policy and using it, the per diem nursing home cost may well double and render the indemnity almost meaningless. But additional long-term care indemnity coverage will be priced according to age.

Assumptions about long-term inflation rates for nursing home and other services are critical in policy analysis. They are difficult to make and open to challenge. A small difference has large effects on total costs and "affordability" by individuals. The Brookings Institution study assumes a 5.8 percent annual nursing home inflation rate, based on historical trends (Rivlin and Wiener, 1988). Since this exceeds the expected rate of improvement in retirement income, the usefulness of a national strategy based primarily on private long-term care insurance of the type described so far is highly questionable. The elderly now spend out of pocket about 12 percent of income on health care, including payment for Medigap insurance. A reasonably good long-term care insurance policy would raise the out-of-pocket spending to over 20 percent of income. The expense is too much for many retirees to handle. According to Robert M. Ball (1989, p. 47), a former U.S. Social Security commissioner, "Most policies advertised as 'inflation protected' are, in short, something far less than that. There is no way [private insurers] can responsibly promise true inflation protection at anything approaching an acceptable price."

Nor does private insurance offer any controls on the prices charged by nursing homes and home care agencies for their services. The indemnity approach insulates the insurer from the control issue. If insurers offered a service benefit in the absence of long-term cost controls, they would be taking an extreme risk. Nursing homes also are unlikely to negotiate such cost limits because of certain imponderables, such as inflation and government reimbursement policy.

Caveat Emptor ("Let the Buyer Beware")

Consumer organizations advise prospective purchasers to investigate the financial stability of the company offering the policy. A number have gone out of business when claims began to be filed. Some companies have sold their long-term care business, and the new owner has raised premiums. Although criteria of the National Association of Insurance Commissioners ask that policies be guaranteed renewable, observing this provision only means that the company cannot cancel the individual's policy. Premiums can be raised for the class of policyholders to which the individual belongs. An increase may be too much for an individual to pay, and the policy will lapse. Switching to a new insurer may be impossible, since the policy-holder is now older and may have acquired conditions that produce unaffordable rates.

Other reasons for wariness are the unfamiliar terms used in the policies and the long history of misrepresentations and other abuses by agents in selling insurance to a population fearful of unpredictable costs. Spokespersons for the industry denounce the relatively few "bad apples" but ask the federal government to stay out of the picture. State insurance departments have been criticized as being weak protectors against the abuses. The problems of abuses and weak state regulation eventually led Congress to reform the Medigap market and might lead it to do likewise in long-term care insurance (see Chapter Five).

Public Policy Questions

From the public policy viewpoint, private long-term care insurance is a doubtful actor in terms of preventing impoverishment, reducing use of Medicaid, and providing stability of coverage (that is, ensuring relatively few lapses in premium payment over time as policyholders age and their financial resources erode). Equally unknown is how well the policies will support independent living in the community or fit into a service spectrum for effective geriatrics.

Forecasts of how much of the older population would buy policies are often discouraging. If 5 percent of income is taken as an indicator of affordability, only about 6 percent of today's elderly could purchase a relatively comprehensive policy. The Brookings Institution estimates that under half the older population in the period 2016–2020 would have private coverage. Assuming even a superior benefits package, the forecasts indicate that relatively few policyholders would escape impoverishment from nursing home expenses.

The policies would pay under 10 percent of long-term care expenses overall. This means that a large proportion of policyholders would have to turn to Medicaid. "A reasonably optimistic estimate would be that by 2016–2020, a third of the elderly could afford a moderately comprehensive freestanding insurance product," the Brookings study found, claiming it used assumptions most favorable to the sale of the insurance (Rivlin and Wiener, 1988, p. 59).

Public Support of Private Insurance

The insurance industry does not argue that private insurance alone can resolve issues of long-term care coverage. The Health Insurance Association of America calls for a combination of public and private action. The public role is to encourage sales to old and young persons through tax favors — such as by deferring taxes through a variant of the Individual Retirement Account for long-term care insurance or through tax deductions for buying the policies. The public role also is to cover through Medicaid those who cannot afford private insurance.

For the long haul, the Health Insurance Association of America foresees mass purchase of long-term care policies by employees. The extent to which employers would make such policies a fringe benefit is problematic. Because employees migrate through various jobs, portability of long-term care insurance reserves built up by employees over the years would have to be provided for.

Though aware of needs for the long-term care coverage, employers are beleaguered by insurance costs for current workers and retirees. A federal task force in the Reagan administration concluded that employers seem unlikely to share the long-term care insurance cost as an added employee benefit in the near future (Task Force on Long-Term Health Care Policies, U.S. Department of Health and Human Services, 1988, p. 44).

The diffidence of younger adults toward protecting themselves against the expenses of long-term care might be overcome if certain conditions were met. These include growth in real income to provide for savings, pensions, and a good living standard. But the possibilities of prefunding a slate of retirement benefits, including retiree health benefits, have not looked as good for workers in general in recent years as they did in the 1960s and early 1970s. Possibilities are dim for labor unions to negotiate for and win group long-term care insurance policies as fringe benefits.

True group policies are rare. In a true group policy, the employer pays part of the premium, every member of the group is covered, and sufficient risk spreading exists to make experience rating of individuals unnecessary. What has been offered through employers are individual policies bought by some and not by others, with medical underwriting and with no financing by the employer. The prices of these "sponsored" policies may be lower because of economies in sales volume. Nonetheless, even in economically good times, sales resistance is high. Younger employees particularly consider need for coverage remote (Polniaszek and Firman, 1991).

Coupling Private Insurance with Medicaid

An attempt has been made to combine private insurance and Medicaid. In this innovation, promoted by the Robert Wood Johnson Foundation, an individual who exhausts private coverage receives Medicaid benefits without being required to meet all or part of a means test. Because of the Medicaid backup, the private insurance can be cheaper. The Medicaid program saves on whatever it would spend for the individual during the insurance period. Presumably, this strategy would appeal to middle-income individuals and deter them from certain spend-down tactics.

An example of this approach is a Connecticut plan. The individual who buys a state-certified policy will receive Medicaid

benefits when the policy benefits are exhausted. The Medicaid
benefits will equal the amount paid under the policy. If the individual purchased a policy with maximum benefit of $100,000
(enough for three years at average prices for nursing homes),
that amount in countable assets would be disregarded when
Medicaid determines eligibility. The asset limit in Connecticut
is $2,000, excluding the value of a home and several other assets.
In effect, the purchaser of the certified policy would have $200,000
worth of nursing home benefits for the price of $100,000. (The
interval covered would vary depending on the rate charged in
the insurance period and the rate—probably lower—charged
in the Medicaid period of the nursing home stay.) This strategy
does nothing to minimize or eliminate application of the Medicaid income test during the Medicaid period of the stay, however. Countable income includes social security, public and private pensions, interest, dividends, net income from property,
rental income, and annuities.

In New York State, where a five-year nursing home stay
may cost up to $335,000, a plan was presented by the state for
certifying policies having these consumer-protection features:
(1) the state would review benefit denials based on disability
status and an appeals board of officials and insurers would ar-
bitrate disputes between policyholders and companies, (2) inflation protection would be at 5 percent compounded, (3) dementia would be covered immediately on purchase and there would
be no social underwriting, (4) minimum benefits would be $100
a day in the nursing home for three years and $50 per day of
home care for six years, (5) a two-month grace period in paying premiums would exist, (6) respite care would be provided
for fourteen days a year, (7) there would be nonforfeiture of
reserves in the event of a federal program for long-term care,
(8) policyholders would have an option to buy more intensive
care coordination than the policy ordinarily provides.

According to James Firman, head of the United Seniors
Health Cooperative, the New York State program had its roots
in the conditions of 1988, when there was no hope of a federal
insurance program and a belief that state government had to
intercede to make private coverage more affordable and depend-

able. More recent political conditions have changed these perspectives, he said.

A dilemma for New York State is that it has the most generous long-term care program under Medicaid in the country, especially for home care, and this generosity makes private insurance less attractive. For example, the community spouse of a nursing home resident may keep $18,000 in income and $70,000 in assets before having to contribute toward care covered by Medicaid. Because of price and medical underwriting, Firman believes that only a minority of older people could buy the certified policies. The state is not guaranteeing real rate stability, according to him. The policies still harbor the potential of large premium increases and high lapse rates. Firman sees 40 cents of every premium dollar going for profit and overhead.

Nonetheless, the state has opened the door to improved private insurance and is working to promote it. A state counseling program for potential buyers of long-term care insurance exists in every county. The state plan offers better consumer protection against unscrupulous agents, obviates the need for asset transfer, and makes it possible to buy a policy with lifetime benefits at the cost of a three-year policy (in effect, a one-third price discount). The state's basic message is that if people will buy a relatively expensive product, the state will make it even better. It is not clear how much the state Medicaid program will save through the program, though it has been estimated at tens of millions of dollars over the long term.

Joshua M. Wiener and Raymond J. Hanley (1992) of the Brookings Institution offer strong objections to this approach. They criticize it as a Medicaid windfall for wealthier individuals who would buy insurance anyway. Medicaid spending would increase because these individuals would be relieved of having to liquidate assets. Both the Connecticut and New York plans assume that asset protection is a key consideration for most people. Yet most older people have under $25,000 in nonhousing assets. Two-thirds have less than $50,000. Moreover, when one study of purchasers asked what their most important reason for buying a policy was, only 14 percent listed asset protection. However, 91 percent of the insurance purchasers said that avoiding Medicaid was their most important reason for buying. The public understands that Medicaid status may not facilitate access to nursing homes because of Medicaid's relatively low payment rates. As Wiener and Hanley (1992, p. 1072) conclude, "Even if all persons turning age 65 in 1992 bought insurance, this population would not become the major part of long-term care users until 2012. A key question, then, is how long are we willing to wait before there are major reforms in how the elderly pay for long-term care?"

To sum up, public and private payment programs — Medicaid, Medicare, Medigap, and indemnity insurance for long-term care — present serious deficiencies in terms of population coverage, comprehensive geriatrics and long-term care, and financial security. How these deficiencies are addressed in proposals for reform is the subject of the next chapter.

7

Politics, Proposals, and Policy Options

What is past is prologue.
— Motto on the National Archives building,
Washington, D.C.

The previous chapters on geriatrics, systems, and payments have taken us through elements of chronic care: professional practice, organized health and social services, and financial structures. In this chapter, we look at proposals for different types of reform: (1) integrated reform of acute and long-term care, (2) long-term care in both institutional and noninstitutional aspects, and (3) long-term home care only. Some reforms focus only on the elderly, and others on all disabled persons. The plans give us perspectives on the continuing debate over the roles government and private insurance should play. An outline of selected proposals is presented in Table 7.1.

Politics and History

A Half-Century of Private Insurance

In the post–World War II period, the federal government's role has been as facilitator to the private sector in the organization and financing of health care. A drive for national health insurance under the Truman administration failed. The goal of improving access to health care was left primarily to labor, management, and insurers, with government covering the poor and the uninsured or uninsurable.

This was epitomized in the 1965 enactment of Medicare and Medicaid. The law made no major changes in the organization of services or in implementing effective limits on provider payments. The expansion of insurance coverage, public and private, increased both the traffic and what it would bear. Predictably, provider charges and costs escalated rapidly.

Access Gives Way to Cost Containment

Efforts to handle costs and access issues together characterized the early 1970s under the Nixon administration. A Democratic proposal for universal, publicly financed and publicly controlled national health insurance was successfully opposed by the health care industry. The focus shifted to federal promotion of health maintenance organizations (HMOs) to resolve cost containment and access problems. After the Nixon-Ford administrations, the Democrats occupied the White House amid hope for a renewed effort for national health insurance. However, impressed by a tax revolt in California, the Carter administration focused on cost containment rather than improved access and lost an attempt to limit hospital costs.

Through the 1980s under Presidents Reagan and Bush, the emphasis was on controlling costs through competition in the health care market. Leaving employers to create their own cost controls, government concentrated on limiting Medicare and Medicaid costs, which contributed to the deficit. Attempts to restrict use of services had little effect on the upward trend in health care costs. All parties tried to save on their respective costs and to fend off cost shifting, but overall costs mounted. The underlying problem was lack of the political clout necessary to force hospitals and physicians to live within a spending ceiling or budget (Davis, 1989).

In industrialized countries with universal coverage and

cost controls, the share of gross domestic product spent on health care averaged a steady 7 percent in the 1980s. This resulted from unified systems of setting or negotiating payments covering all patients (Davis, 1989).

But in the United States, the share was approaching 13 percent, contributing to what business observers thought were American price disadvantages on the world market. The recession of the late 1980s led some employers to reduce or eliminate coverage, and the ranks of the uninsured and underinsured swelled. Weak government revenues were confronted by competing claims for government resources for the uninsured and poorly insured, including a growing number of AIDS patients.

In this context, despite heightened public awareness of long-term care problems, the chances of enacting any major proposal for direct federal payment for services were slim, particularly when the White House thought there was too much government interference in American life.

Policy conflicts over long-term care mirrored basic divisions between advocates of bigger and lesser government. A task force in the Reagan administration endorsed a government role to facilitate the small but growing market for private long-term care insurance (discussed in Chapter Six). The strategy assumed that the "successes" of regular health insurance could be duplicated in the long-term care field.

The task force advocated tax incentives for purchase of private policies by individuals and job-based groups, regulation to guard against insurance abuses, and efforts to educate people on their responsibility to protect themselves against long-term care costs. For the poor, there would still be Medicaid, a continuing drain on federal and state treasuries.

Proposals for comprehensive benefits financed by social insurance and other taxes were put forward by the late Representative Claude Pepper (D-Fla.) and other Democrats. Fiscal issues prompted the design of proposals for young and old, some for the elderly only (at least at the start), and some for home and community-based care only. The roles for Medicaid and private insurance were sharply limited.

This strategy takes the view that the problem cannot be

solved by the private sector and that access to long-term care must be universal without tests of ability to pay. While this country has never put into law the idea that access to health care is a right, the social insurance point of view verges on this position. It contrasts with the notion that health care is a "product" dispensed through a market based on ability to pay, with exceptional procedures for the poor.

A Reagan-Bush administration attempt to curry favor with older voters through a minor and relatively inexpensive improvement in Medicare's hospitalization benefit mushroomed in the hands of a Democratic Congress into a major expansion of Medicare: the Medicare Catastrophic Coverage Act of 1988. But Congress held back on long-term care. This act, however, authorized the Bipartisan Commission on Comprehensive Health Care to consider both regular and long-term care.

To win White House approval, funding for the complex program — including a costly outpatient drug benefit — was placed largely on the shoulders of the wealthier Medicare beneficiaries rather than on payroll taxpayers of all ages. Groups of outspoken beneficiaries demanded repeal, and Congress acquiesced. The episode dimmed the chances for imminent long-term care legislation.

Surviving the ill-fated law were the commission (whose results are reviewed later in this chapter) and provisions to ease the "spousal impoverishment" problem (discussed in Chapter Five). Medicaid remained the principal program financing long-term care, and nursing home costs remained a threat to state budgets.

States looked for ways to draw more federal funding. They developed the tactic of taxing providers to raise the state part of the Medicaid fiscal match. States also wanted flexibility in how they organized and financed services. For example, states considered how to mix or pool various kinds of funding and how to substitute home and community-based care for nursing home care.

Private insurance seemed to some states to be a promising way to ease Medicaid spending on long-term care. With foundation support, several states have considered offering Medicaid benefits proportionate to the purchase of private long-term care insurance, an option examined in Chapter Six.

Budget pressures stimulated innovative thinking at the state level, consonant with geriatrics' views. The National Governors' Association in 1986 called for development of a continuing care system with a single entry point and case management (care coordination). It also sought pooled funding involving Medicaid and Medicare and capacity to innovate in the direction of state-sponsored social and health maintenance organizations linking acute and long-term care.

Federal policy appeared to be splintered. Federal agencies conducted policy-related research into long-term care issues. Congress encouraged experiments and demonstrations in the organization and funding of long-term care under Medicare, Medicaid, and other government programs. But federal austerity measures narrowed the use of the Medicare home care benefit, particularly making certain none of it went for long-term care. Beneficiaries went to court and won cases over alleged illegal administrative decisions.

Groups representing older people, disabled people, Alzheimer's disease patients, and the poor became more vocal about long-term care. Television journalism depicted health and long-term care problems, making Americans vividly aware that Medicare did not cover long-term care and that Medicaid did not prevent destitution.

The presidential election of 1992 brought in a Democratic administration committed to change in health and long-term care. President Clinton clearly linked deficit reduction, control of health costs, and economic revival as prime objectives of his administration.

Proposals and Options

The proposals described in Table 7.1 illustrate the range of options available to the White House and Congress. Some proposals represent a complex mix of options. For example, some combine public insurance, private insurance, public assistance, and out-of-pocket spending. The proposals also represent

Table 7.1. Proposals for Long-Term Care Reform.

	Population Covered	Pocketbook Relief	Service Spectrum	Cost to Government	Main Financing	Administration
Public						
Comprehensive	All	Higher	All	Higher	Taxes	Fed-St
Harvard	Medicare	Medium	Mcr/LTC	Medium	SI	Fed
Pepper Commission	All	Medium	LTC	Medium	Taxes	Fed-St
Mitchell Bill	Elderly	Medium	Home + NH after 2 years	Medium	SI + PI	Fed-St-Pvt
Kennedy Bill	All	Medium	Home + 6 mos. NH	Medium	SI	Fed-St[a]
Medicare Part C	Medicare	Higher	All	Higher	Medicare	Fed
Commonwealth	Poor 65+	Higher	All	Lower	Medicare	Fed
Mixed						
Governors	Medicare Medicaid	Medium	All	Medium	Medicare Medicaid[b]	St-Fed
Private						
HHS Task Force	Buyers	Unclear[c]	LTC	Lower	Premiums	Insurers + IRS[d]

Note: LTC = Long-term care
NH = Nursing home
Home = Home care
Fed = Federal
St = State
IRS = Internal Revenue Service

[a]Individual has opportunity to buy into federal insurance program covering nursing home stays beyond six months.

[b]Possibility of Medicaid tie-in with private insurance.

[c]Pocketbook relief of premium payment depends on income of buyer and quality of options picked. For most older people, relief is low, especially if policy has an inflation adjustment. Pocketbook relief for individual receiving services may be high until benefits are exhausted. However, if benefit has not been adjusted for inflation (requiring higher premium), the pocketbook relief may be low during period of care.

[d]Policy would have to meet federal criteria to qualify for tax deduction.

different approaches to program administration and service organization.

The basic question of how much change is necessary is a matter of judgment as well as knowledge. Does the country need only minor adjustments within the current structure of long-term care, including access, organization, delivery, and financing? Or are fundamental reforms needed? What can realistically be expected of private insurance and of government at the state and federal levels?

What seems beyond dispute is that doing nothing to change current policy will allow total spending for long-term care, including federal spending under current law, to rise rapidly. The reasons are the aging of the baby-boom generation, improvements in life expectancy, and likely rates of price increase above general inflation.

As the Congressional Budget Office (1991) put it, "Financing long-term care (LTC) services presents policymakers with a dilemma because the various goals of policy that many see as desirable are inherently inconsistent. In particular, containing the burgeoning total costs of LTC that are anticipated under current policies conflicts with providing better protection for LTC users against the out-of-pocket costs of this care, broadening the range of services available, and improving their quality."

If the policymaker is most concerned about the level and growth of federal long-term care costs, the option of relying on the private sector for a larger financing role is obviously desirable. The policymaker who emphasizes financial protection for people and a broader range and higher quality of services is opting necessarily for increased total spending for long-term care, probably including far more federal spending than contemplated under current law.

The relationship of long-term care to acute care is often omitted in policy analyses. When both realms are considered together, options are possible for transferring savings across sectors. If, as some critics contend, 25 percent of U.S. health care spending represents waste, this is enough money to fill the gaps and provide all the health and long-term care Americans need.

Capturing that alleged waste may take time, ingenuity, and courage in the face of providers, insurers, and others with livelihoods at stake.

Harvard Medicare Project

A collaboration of physicians, economists, and political scientists, this project offered a plan to extend Medicare into long-term care and preventive medicine. It also aimed to develop administrative structures that would unify the spectrum of services and simplify access by patients and families. At the same time, the project sought to control the rapid escalation of the costs of formal care and to limit what patients and families had to pay out of pocket at time of service need.

The expanded Medicare would provide for long-term care in the nursing home and the community, subject to a geriatrics assessment (discussed in Chapters Three and Four). Medicare would cover the cost of an annual physical examination limited to specified screening tests, such as Pap smear and tests of blood pressure, serum cholesterol, and stool, and a rectal examination.

To control costs as well as to provide unified patient management, Medicare would encourage enrollment in HMOs. At the same time, over a five- to ten-year period, Medicare would place aggregate spending for doctor services in an area on an annual budget. All doctors would take assignment—that is, they could not charge the patient more than the Medicare-recognized fee for a service.

Meanwhile, Medicare would authorize states to determine a budget for all Medicare hospital services within their borders. Each hospital would negotiate a limit with the state on what Medicare would pay that hospital.

Financing the expanded coverage would be a mixture of payroll taxes, premiums, and general revenues. Nursing home patients would contribute 80 percent of their monthly social security benefit as a residential copayment. There also would be a one-month deductible.

All elders would pay Medicare premiums on an income-related, not flat, basis. A surtax equal to 5 percent of the income tax would be paid by the 40 percent of elders who pay income taxes. States would have to buy Medicare coverage for all elders with incomes below 125 percent of the federal poverty line.

No beneficiary would have to spend more than $1,000 a year in Medicare copayments. Annual premiums would be raised an additional $150 to $200 per beneficiary, and beneficiaries as a whole would be responsible for 25 percent of program costs. The hospital deductible would be halved, the physician deductible eliminated, and the physician coinsurance cut to 10 percent from 20 percent.

The Medicare long-term care addition was estimated to reach $50 billion a year (in 1985 dollars) within ten years of implementation. About $35 billion would replace Medicaid and out-of-pocket spending.

The authors of the project argued against private insurance. They said it would not work: few people would buy long-term care coverage before reaching the ages at which they are likely to need it. By then, private policies are too expensive. Fearing overuse of services, insurers will offer less than a full range of noninstitutional care or price the coverage expensively. Marketing costs make policies even more costly and less affordable.

Private Insurance with Federal Support

A Congressionally authorized task force on long-term care was appointed in 1986 by the Reagan administration to examine the development of private insurance. The role of state and federal governments was considered. The task force report, issued in 1987, was seen as a tool for heading off Medicare expansion into long-term care just at the time Congress was considering coverage of catastrophic expenses under Medicare (Task Force on Long-Term Health Care Policies, U.S. Department of Health and Human Services, 1987). The task force called for tax incentives to encourage sales of private insurance. Because they would mean revenue losses and enlarge the federal deficit, the recommendations were controversial within the Reagan White House.

The greatest potential for covering large numbers of people, the panel said, was through employer sponsorship and pension funds. Federal and state tax codes should encourage the purchase of insurance "without unduly reducing government revenues." For example, the codes should be modified to permit favorable tax treatment of reserves and interest built up by long-term care insurance accounts. The codes should allow individuals to make tax-free transfers among retirement income instruments such as pensions and annuities to facilitate purchase of the insurance.

The panel aimed at moving insurance away from acute care orientations. For example, in determining eligibility for long-term care benefits, insurers should consider using ADLs instead of "medical necessity" criteria. Insurers should avoid making coverage for institutional services depend on distinctions among skilled nursing, intermediate care, and custodial services.

Among forty-one recommendations, the task force also called for government efforts to inform consumers about their need for protection against the costs of long-term care and efforts to protect consumers against sales abuses and inadequate insurance coverages. Government and insurers should collaborate in collecting and sharing long-term care data. In covering home and community care as well as nursing home care, the panel wanted insurers to have latitude to experiment with benefit design, utilization controls, and care coordination.

Pepper Commission

In 1988, a special commission — the Bipartisan Commission on Comprehensive Health Care — was established by the president and Congressional leaders. It was renamed the Pepper Commission after Claude D. Pepper (D-Fla.), its first chair, died in 1989. Senator John D. Rockefeller IV (D-W.Va.) took over as chair. Among its tasks was to make a report and recommendations on long-term care as well as on covering uninsured persons for medical and hospital benefits.

Its recommendations on the uninsured were approved by a vote of eight to seven, but those on long-term care did far better, eleven to four. The highlights of the plan are as follows:

1. Long-term care systems under a social insurance program, with users paying 20 percent of cost (actual or average).
2. Protection of beneficiaries against impoverishment by
   a. Home care expenses through social insurance with coinsurance (20 percent of actual cost or of a national average cost).
   b. Nursing home expenses, covered under social insurance (with users paying 20 percent) for the first three months and a liberalized Medicaid-type program afterward.
3. Private insurance — to fill gaps in the plan — encouraged by certain tax advantages, meeting minimum federal standards, and enforced by the states to prevent misrepresentation and sales abuses. (States should educate the public about long-term care insurance.)
4. Benefits for individuals with at least three ADL deficiencies or cognitive impairment (determined by assessment) and prescribed in a care plan. The plan is developed by professionals and the family and is carried out with help from a care coordinator, who could authorize payments for services pursuant to certain ceilings (for example, home care up to the cost of nursing home care).
5. Administration under federal contract by states, which designate local agencies to supervise assessments, care planning, and care coordination, to certify service providers, and to establish a review and appeals process. Federal standards and guidelines cover standardized assessment criteria, certification of assessment agencies, guidelines for certifying care coordinators, care manager budgets, and provider payment rates.
6. Research and development to prevent or delay the need for institutionalization, to manage care, to perfect the delivery and integration of services, to develop outcome measures and practice guidelines, and examine the special problems of
   a. Disadvantaged racial and ethnic minorities.
   b. The rural elderly.
   c. The nonelderly disabled.
   Funded gradually to reach $1 billion a year by the federal government.

Had the long-term care plan been in full swing in 1990, the cost would have been $42.8 billion for the year (Table 7.2). This is described as "net new federal cost"—that is, cost above what govenrment spent in 1990 (chiefly under Medicare and Medicaid). The plan rebalances long-term care in favor of noninstitutional services. Institutionally, the plan invests heavily in convalescence and rehabilitation by covering all the costs of short nursing home stays. Nursing home entrants having long stays (over three months) would be financed only marginally by the plan; their mainstay after out-of-pocket spending would be Medicaid, liberalized by the plan (Figure 7.1).

The plan concentrates on low-income people, not the relatively wealthy (Figure 7.2); three-quarters of beneficiaries would be at 150 percent or less of the federal poverty level. The plan exemplifies programs like social security: framed (and paid for) universally and giving a substantial boost to people at common income levels.

The plan would save individuals and families $6.9 billion in out-of-pocket expenses for nursing home care, or $3,000 per user. Many of these people would have spent down to Medicaid. Some two million disabled elders would use home

Table 7.2. Beneficiaries and Net Federal Costs of Pepper Commission Long-Term Care Recommendations, by Age Group and Type of Service.

	Home care	Nursing home care	Total
Total beneficiaries (in millions)			
Elderly	2.0	1.2	3.2
Nonelderly	1.0	.2	1.2
Total	3.0	1.4	4.4
New federal costs (in billions, 1990)			
Elderly	$15.0	$16.8	$31.8
Nonelderly	9.0	2.0	11.0
Total	$24.0	$18.8	$42.8

Source: Pepper Commission, 1990, p. 130.

Figure 7.1. How Elderly Nursing Home Entrants Benefit from
Pepper Commission Plan, Compared with Current Law.

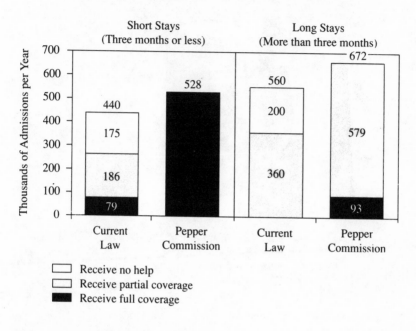

Source: Pepper Commission, 1990.

care, double the current number using paid care. For the one
million disabled elders who now buy home care, savings would
equal $900 million, or about $1,000 per user. The program
would serve 4.4 million persons, including 1.2 million nonelderly
persons. Three million persons would receive home care (totaling
$24 billion) and 1.4 million, nursing home care (totaling $18.8
billion).

The recommendations for the uninsured and for long-term
care carried no specific financing plan, an omission that some
friends and foes of the commission considered a fault. But specific financing proposals might have upset the small majority
of commission members who favored the plan for the uninsured
as well as the large majority who supported long-term care.

The commission did offer options from which to compose
a financing plan, though. The choice, the Pepper report declared,

Figure 7.2. Number of Beneficiaries of Pepper Commission
Long-Term Care Plan, by Income Relative to Federal Poverty Level.

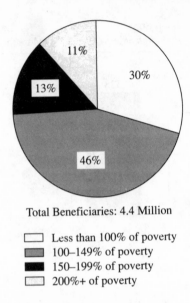

Total Beneficiaries: 4.4 Million

☐ Less than 100% of poverty
▨ 100–149% of poverty
■ 150–199% of poverty
☐ 200%+ of poverty

Source: Pepper Commission, 1990.

should be guided by these criteria: (1) progressive taxes; (2) contributions required of everyone; (3) revenue yields that keep up with benefit growth, estimated at 9 percent per year. Under a four-year phasing schedule, costs (in 1990 dollars) would be as follows: $10.8 billion, $25.0 billion, $32.8 billion, and $42.8 billion.

The commission report also included a recommendation to expand Medicare at an estimated 1990 cost of $200 million to cover colorectal and prostate screening and other cost-effective preventive measures. With mammography and Pap smears, these provisions would have moved Medicare well into preventive medicine.

Comprehensive Social Insurance

Among the most comprehensive proposals for a federally based long-term care program was one by the American Association of Retired Persons, Older Women's League, and Villers Foundation (now Families USA) in the late 1980s.

Elders as well as other adults and children would be covered, mainly through social security. Services would be available on the basis of need for care, as evaluated by a local care coordination agency using a comprehensive protocol. A full range of institutional and noninstitutional services would be provided. The details included help with home and financial management, home adjustment equipment, minor home and vehicle modification, and protective services. Coupled to state administration under federal guidelines and joint funding would be the use of public or private nonprofit organizations as the local agencies. They would contract with for-profit and nonprofit providers to deliver services. It would be up to the states to certify the agencies and providers, define allowable costs, monitor quality, train administrators and practitioners, and designate representatives on quality control councils and boards. The agencies would have teams of professionals trained in social and health needs of the chronically ill. The agencies would work closely with housing authorities and Medicare. Demonstration programs of service delivery and payment would be conducted.

Financing for the program would come from such options as payroll taxes, estate taxes, an additional Medicare premium paid by elders (except for the poor), deductibles, and federal-state general revenues equal to current Medicaid spending on long-term care. Private insurers would be encouraged to provide coverage of copays, deductibles, and uncovered services as well as of alternative living arrangements, such as in assisted-living facilities.

A congressionally named commission would advise on technical, payment, implementation, and other issues. The program would be phased in over two years. Administrative and service delivery systems would be developed by the states under planning grants. In the third and fourth years, home and community services would be activated. In the fourth year, nursing home care would be covered. By that time, there would be coordinated long-term care networks in the states. Medicaid and state-only funding programs would have been merged into the new program.

Carve-Out Proposals

A lower price tag can be achieved by carving out large functions for private insurance from the matrix of a comprehensive social insurance program. Home and community-based services would remain a government responsibility, but nursing home care would be shared with the private insurance. People would receive a needs assessment from a care coordinating agency under public auspices. If nursing home placement was advised, according to a proposal by Senator George Mitchell (D-Maine), people would use private insurance designed for the first two years, after which the government program would cover expenses. If they did not have private insurance, they would be faced with $50,000 or more of expense for the two years. Few persons could cover this expense without having to seek help from Medicaid.

Because very long nursing home stays would fall to government coverage, insurers presumably would be able and willing to design less expensive policies (including other services besides the first two nursing home years) and presumably would attract a larger clientele. Favorable tax treatment would be provided for premiums paid for the private coverage. This may do little for certain groups, however. First, individuals already old or disabled would probably be excluded from coverage because of medical underwriting and age-related pricing. A large role would remain for Medicaid programs, compromising the role of social insurance as a first-line protector against impoverishment. This kind of carve-out contradicts the social insurance goal of serving all income levels and offering low-income contributors more in relation to their contributions than higher-income contributors, according to Robert M. Ball, a former Social Security commissioner. The carve-out turns that principle on its head. "Workers would have to contribute to a long-term care protection program that would not in fact protect them," he comments (Ball, 1989, p. 94). Second, if made a deductible expense rather than a credit, the tax treatment would be useless to lower-income taxpayers. Third, the strategy depends on the quality of the coverage, stability of the insurer, the effect of inflation, and the absence of lapses in premium payment.

Fourth, the strategy accepts expenses that would not occur under social insurance, such as sales expense and the higher per capita costs of administration.

For the variant in which the government program pays for the first year, the role for private insurance is to cover the longer nursing home stay. As envisioned by Ball, this approach protects the individual's income and assets as long as the spouse needs them or for possible return to the community. After a year in as a nursing home resident, Ball says, the individual is likely to be a permanent resident. If the resident has a community-living spouse, the social insurance coverage continues. But if not, it then becomes reasonable to apply income and assets to the costs of the nursing home, with a small reserve for personal needs. The protection of a legacy is a doubtful high priority for a public program, he says. Besides, individuals seeking to protect a legacy may have the means to buy private insurance. Otherwise, they should be covered by an improved Medicaid program.

The purpose of the "before" or "after" carve-out is to reduce the expense of a public program. The "before" variation, as proposed by Senator Mitchell in 1987, would have an estimated cost of $16 to $18 billion a year, counting a deductible, premium, and copayments. The "after" variation, says Ball, will reduce the public cost of long-term care substantially — by at least one-third — as compared to a plan with unrestricted nursing home coverage. Ball estimated an unrestricted plan at $50 billion in 1990 (or 1 percent of payroll contributed by employees and 1 percent by employers). Since the proposed program would absorb expenses paid by other programs, its net additional cost would be $20 billion. If only the net increase were to be financed for sixty years, Ball (1989, pp. 69–99) says, this would require adding about 0.75 percent to the social security contribution rate of employees and the same to the employer rate.

Senator Kennedy proposed a bill with optional federal insurance for the period beyond the first six nursing home months. Besides the short-term nursing home benefit and covered home and community-based services for elders, other disabled adults, and children, this proposal calls for individuals to elect federal long-term nursing home insurance at age forty-five or at age sixty-five, paying premiums related to age at issue of policy. Under Kennedy's Lifecare Insurance Program, Senate bill 2681 of 1988, the optional federal insurance could not be purchased by individuals already in a nursing home or who had been patients there in the sixty days prior to signing up for coverage. Premium rates would be set federally, and a 35 percent per diem copayment would be required.

The Kennedy plan was estimated at $20.5 billion annual in new spending. States would make contributions to the program equal to savings it would produce for Medicaid. The total included $9 billion for home and community care, $10 billion for six months of nursing home care, and $1.5 billion as the tax-subsidized portion of the $4.5 billion optional insurance program. The senator said financing could be arranged by making higher earnings subject to the Social Security/Medicare payroll tax and by adjusting alcohol and tobacco excises.

The legislation is noteworthy for authorizing grants (no amount set) for training professional persons in home and community-based care, for training home aides, for consumer education, and for long-term care planning and technical assistance. Also noteworthy is the unique provision of the Ball plan to assign 0.05 percent of the social security contributions to research on age-related diseases, yielding about $1.4 billion in 1990.

Pepper Home Care Bill, 1988

A bill that contains no provisions for nursing home coverage — and therefore was estimated to cost under $6 billion a year averaged over five years — was proposed by the late Representative Claude Pepper. Designed to force a vote on the issue of long-term care benefits before the 1988 elections, the bill called for expanding Medicare to provide home care for chronically ill adults and children unable to perform two or more ADLs.

The home care benefits include nursing, homemaker/ home health assistance, medical social services, and physical and other therapies. Financing would be through extension of the Social Security/Medicare payroll tax to higher incomes. Recipients of benefits would have a copayment of up to 5 percent of costs if the tax proved inadequate, thus guaranteeing that the program would not add to the federal deficit. Benefits would be managed through independent state and local government agencies using care coordinators. Aiming to complement family care, the bill would provide training, counseling, and respite to families.

Medicare (Part C)

In 1987, Representatives Pepper and Edward Roybal (D-Calif.) introduced the Comprehensive Catastrophic Health Insurance Act, designed not only to cover long-term care but also to fill other gaps in Medicare — sufficient to transform it into a geriatrics program. The bill would add a Part C to Medicare. It would provide certain preventive care and health promotion benefits, eliminate copayments for doctor and hospital care, cover unlimited hospital stays, cover outpatient drugs, hearing, eye and dental services, and provide comprehensive long-term care managed by geriatrics specialists.

More than that, the bill would develop contracts between Medicare and organizations of providers, insurers, and others to provide the Part C package and standard Medicare benefits under a capitated rate. Financing would come from usual Medicare payments, payments for private Medigap policies, Part B premiums, state and federal Medicaid payments for services absorbed by Part C, and revenues from improving the tax base for Medicare.

Savings were expected from more sensible and efficient management of services paid by Medicare. States would be required to buy Part C for Medicaid-eligible beneficiaries. The program would absorb $20 billion in Medicaid nursing home expenses and receive about $40 billion in payroll taxes in addition to beneficiary payments.

Commonwealth Fund Commission

Medicare should be expanded to cover home care and adult day care for 1.6 million elders (called "severely impaired") who have two or more ADL deficiencies and require assistance from another person. Putting long-term care within Medicare should facilitate integration of medical and long-term care needs.

The expansion should build on privately paid and Medicaid-financed services. It should promote the development and operation of high-quality, accountable, and comprehensive chronic care services in every community. Eligibility should be determined by a comprehensive assessment of physical and cognitive functioning. Families should be helped with care planning and management. Quality standards, including training requirements for home care workers, would be set and monitored.

Benefits include fifteen to twenty-five hours a week of in-home personal care. Two hours of adult day care could be substituted for each hour of in-home care. Beneficiaries would buy more care. Families could determine the service configuration. The plan carries a 20 percent cost-sharing provision. However, for low-income impaired elders, Medicaid should help cover cost sharing and supplementary benefits on a sliding scale of contributions. About 1.3 million of the 1.6 severely impaired elders have incomes below 200 percent of the federal poverty level.

Private insurance should be expanded to cover cost sharing under Medicare and in-home care for less severely impaired elders able to buy private protection.

After deducting $1.7 billion in Medicaid savings, the cost would have been $6.8 billion in 1989, or, in the year 2000, when the affected population would reach 2.1 million, a net cost of $9.3 billion (after deducting Medicaid savings of $2.4 billion). The assessment component alone would have been $100 million in 1989 and administration $800 million (Commonwealth Fund Commission on Elderly People Living Alone, 1989).

Constructing a Program

Other options can be developed from elements of the foregoing proposals in order to fit various political and fiscal requirements. In preparing its health care reforms, the Clinton administration considered benefit and financing patterns seen in those proposals. Given an administration wary of the politics and costs of the federal deficit as well as taxpayer burdens, what kinds of options would appear most practical? The following presents possible answers to this question.

Lower-Cost Federal Options for Long-Term Care

1. Incremental Medicaid reform
    A. Through the home and community-based waiver or block grants to states willing to participate in improving noninstitutional care.
    B. Liberalized test of income and assets to qualify for nursing home care (and tight restrictions on asset transfers).
    C. Improved regulation of private long-term care insurance, provision of limited tax incentives to promote sales, and coordination with Medicaid (along lines of the New York State program described in Chapter Six).
    D. Cost to federal government: $5 billion in FY 1994.
2. Low-income program of home and community-based services
    A. Improved retention of income and assets for nursing home residents under Medicaid.
    B. Block grant program for mentally retarded/developmentally disabled persons.
    C. Work incentives for the disabled, with tax credits up to half of personal assistance services (maximum $15,000).
    D. Voluntary *public* insurance covering up to $30,000 in expenses; one-time chance to buy at age sixty-five, and five-year waiting period before benefits would be paid under the plan. (This arrangement leaves gaps to be filled by private insurance.)
    E. Improved regulation of private insurance and provision of limited tax incentives.
    F. Cost to federal government: $7 billion in FY 1994.
3. Home and community-based services through social insurance (payroll tax)

A. Covers all people with severe disabilities, without regard to income, with entitlement to assessment, plan of care, and services on a funds-available basis (with sliding scale of fees for services).

B. Financing capped by global budget.

C. Premium like that of Medicare Part B (paid by program participants, except for the poor) of $20 monthly to offset federal costs.

D. Block grants to the states to cover mentally retarded/developmentally disabled persons.

E. Residual Medicaid program, with liberalized income and asset limits.

F. Cost to federal government: $15.4 billion in FY 1994.

G. Possible integration with service benefits under Department of Veterans Affairs and with health maintenance organizations.

4. Complete coverage through social insurance

A. Home and community-based services and nursing home care are covered.

B. Cost to federal government: $6 billion in FY 1994 (rising to $126 billion in 2020).

C. Possible integration with service benefits under Department of Veterans Affairs and with health maintenance organizations.

D. Sixteen-year phase-in period

   i.   Costs rise from $6 billion for a restricted program starting in 1994 to $93 billion for a full program in 2010, thence to $126 billion ten years later with retirements of baby boomers.

   ii. The initial program in 1994 would cover (a) home care for severely disabled persons at or below the federal poverty level and (b) nursing home care under a liberalized Medicaid asset limits. At intervals, the income and asset limits are eased; social insurance displaces Medicaid for nursing home care by 2010, with residents paying a 20 percent coinsurance.

The outlined options vary in estimated first-year costs from $5 billion to $15 billion. The option with the highest ultimate costs (Option 4) has a phase-in period of sixteen years (1994–2010), with an estimate of the succeeding decade to show the impact on costs of the baby-boom cohort. Provision is made for private as well as public voluntary insurance.

Conclusion

There is a rich supply of ideas for organizing and financing long-term care and creating bridges to acute care. Approaches range from those funded solely through social insurance or through private insurance and those that combine elements of both plus public assistance (Medicaid). The choice of approach lies in one's values, knowledge, and judgments, and how much one is willing to compromise for the sake of a working program — imperfect but attainable in the near future rather than in never-never land. There is not so much a dearth of ideas and program models as a dearth of will to decide. We are all open to the risk of long-term disability and we are all getting older. For those reasons alone our country has to be willing to take a chance.

A sense of history may be helpful in determining our future. How has our society changed and what do the trends tell us? We should take into account the socioeconomic, health status, and demographic changes over the last half century as well as our experience with the political, financial, and administrative dynamics of private insurance, public insurance, and public assistance. Our final chapter takes the plunge, offering the author's recommendations on what to do.

8

Within Our Grasp: Long-Term Care Security

The issue of the cost of long-term care actually poses the most dire consequences over the long range for the Baby Boom generation, "sandwiched" in the middle of child care, elder care, and other competing demands, and faced with their own long-term care risks and needs in the future.
— Executive Office on Aging, Office of the Governor, State of Hawaii, 1991, p. 9-3

In this chapter, we counter some arguments against a long-term care plan, review the reasons why one is urgently needed, and offer concrete recommendations. This chapter deals with some of the issues that will figure in Congressional deliberations of President Clinton's plans.

Attempts to introduce a broad long-term care program face several hurdles: the notion that it is a frill, that the problem is intractable, that a plan should wait until acute care costs are contained, and that private insurance and Medicaid are enough, with adjustments.

There is also a question of linkage to economic prospects. The President has tied health reform to improvement of the federal deficit and the economy. Questions have been raised about how much the country can safely absorb in new taxes or mandated costs for health reform as well as for deficit control. The

122

President has argued that the deficit has created pressures for bold reform, while opponents of strong government action say the deficit requires small steps. Although there is widespread public insecurity about regular health coverage and long-term care, there appears to be a limited willingness to accept higher taxes. Public confidence in government, especially the President, will help determine whether these conditions play out in favor of comprehensive change or not. The likelihood is that any proposal for reform of the health care economy, which amounts to one-seventh of the total U.S. economy, will move slowly enough through Congress to become an issue in another election. Historians will note a contrast with the last time major federal health legislation was enacted: a Democratic president (Lyndon Johnson) was elected by an enormous landslide, had a huge majority in Congress, and had a growing economy.

Making the Case for Long-Term Care

The White House has ample evidence to marshal for reforms affecting long-term care. It can look to states like Florida, Hawaii, and New York on long-term care needs. Evidence contradicting the notions given above has been presented in this book. There is far more that could be said, but what we have presented may be enough to show the necessity and urgency of meeting America's long-term care needs. The issues can be solved.

The tractability of the issues is clear to officials of the state of Hawaii, which happens to have its own form of national health insurance. A 1991 report to the governor and legislature concluded that "it is possible for a State, and certainly for the nation, to provide affordable protection from the dramatically rising costs of long term care to a broad range of individuals and families." The report added that "it is simply a matter of time before elder care overtakes child care as a priority employment issue with clear ramifications for the productivity and well-being of employees and for the profitability of any business." The existence of reliable financing for long-term care was viewed as a precondition for the development of an adequate infrastructure of services and workers (Executive Office on Aging, Office of the Governor, State of Hawaii, 1991, pp. 9-2, 9-3).

The Argument for Cost Containment

This book has argued that the organization and financing of long-term care are essential to a balanced health care system. Grounds also exist for arguing that the resolution of long-term care issues will assist the reform of acute care in achieving the goals of universal access, comprehensive benefits, and cost containment.

Long-term care is a key to cost containment in a health care economy approaching $1 trillion a year. Chapters Three and Four carried the message that people with chronic disability need and use, where it exists, a continuum of services.

How hospital and other acute care costs can be restrained when there is a vigorous long-term care program in the system can be seen in Manitoba, the Canadian province we visited in Chapter Four. Because of a sputtering economy and reductions in federal aid, Manitoba could not delay cost constraints but needed a way to do it without compromising a commitment to universal access to comprehensive benefits. A major basis of the Manitoba strategy is a shift toward equally effective and lower-cost health services. This means allocating resources based on cost-effectiveness: Does the investment actually produce a desirable result worth the money spent on it? Are there choices to be made between high-cost and low-cost effective procedures, institutions, and patterns of service?

U.S. studies have shown that, in adjacent areas, different styles of treating a given disease sometimes show large differences in expense but little or no difference in treatment outcome. The key to economizing on health care in the United States can be the elimination of services of marginal value and the provision of care in equally effective but lower-cost ways. The techniques of outcome study can be applied to verifying that changes in service delivery actually benefit patients, such as shifting the site of care for certain patients from the expensive hospital to the less expensive personal care home (nursing home) and home of the patient, supported by home care and community services.

In 1992, Manitoba began doing exactly that. "Common sense would tell us that if we expand our programs of home care so that these services are available to many more people in Manitoba who might otherwise have had to be hospitalized or have had to stay in hospital longer, the incidence of hospitalization and/or the average length of hospital stay should go down and hospital and total health care costs should be contained," the government declares (Manitoba Health Department, 1992, p. 17).

"If we close one urban community-hospital bed, we can open seven personal care [nursing home] beds or serve 25 people on home care or include over 225 seniors in support service projects in the community or in senior [age-segregated] housing," commented Betty Havens, assistant deputy minister, Continuing Care Programs Division, Manitoba Health Department (personal communication, March 1993).

The plan recognizes that health care expenditures originate outside the formal provision of services. Consequently, emphasis is put on activities of health promotion, disability postponement, disease prevention, and the education of citizens to make informed decisions (Figure 8.1). The plan asks for the user's attention, not out-of-pocket supplements (a typical ploy in the cost-shifting patterns found in the United States).

The plan calls on service providers to consolidate services for the sake of economy and to be flexible in meeting the needs of Manitobans, which can change.

Unified Planning and Payment

This strategy is possible because there is a single payer for comprehensive services: the provincial government. With just one year into the effort, inflation has been zero instead of double digits, and $26 million has been saved in an annual budget of $1.9 billion for provincial health. This kind of cost control would be comparable to saving almost $100 billion in 1992 U.S. health care costs. This strategy of less reliance on hospitals is feasible not only because Manitoba has a relatively well-developed program of home and community-based care, but also because, as noted, there is a single payer, the provincial government. There is hardly any commercial insurance, or the need for it.

Figure 8.1. Conception of an Organized Continuum of Services (After Manitoba Health Department).

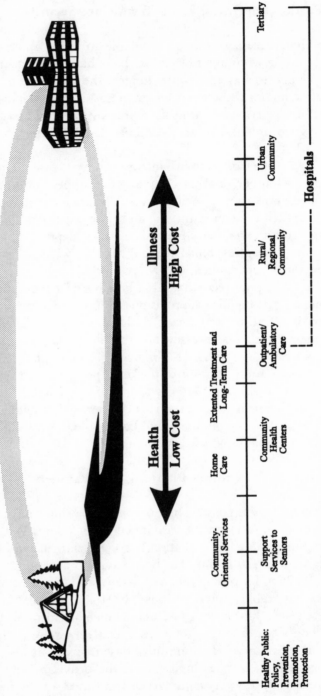

Hospital / Community   Community / Hospital

Health   Illness
Low Cost   High Cost

Healthy Public: Community-   Home   Extended Treatment and   Outpatient/   Rural/   Urban   Tertiary
Policy,   Oriented Services Care   Long-Term Care   Ambulatory   Regional   Community
Prevention,   Support Services   Community   Care   Community
Promotion,   to Seniors   Health
Protection   Centers

                                                                                  ———— Hospitals ————

Source: Manitoba Health Department, 1992, p. 13.

The Manitoba effort is not unique. British Columbia, too, has a managed system of health and long-term care. The long-term care system is designed to support care provided by the family and other informal caregivers. As an official of the provincial health department puts it, "Whatever its shortcomings, as the Canadian long-term care system evolves, the concept of an integrated delivery system for acute and long-term care offers a society an enhanced opportunity for making sound decisions on how best to meet the needs of its citizens at an affordable cost. In Canada, these decisions are made in partnership among government, provider and individual. From our perspective, our health systems seem less adversarial and more cooperative than those of the United States. Perhaps that's just the nature of the Canadian people" (Pallan, 1993, p. 112).

We have seen in Chapter Four that some U.S. programs combine acute and long-term care under a single administration, using pooled payments from public and private sources. However, these are scattered projects and cover a minuscule part of the population in need of long-term care services. It is conceivable, if not likely, though, that these projects could prosper and proliferate through financing of the service spectrum through a single payer or a group of payers under a common set of rules authorized by government.

In pursuing a long-term care strategy consonant with cost containment, there could be a role for private insurance. But such a role should probably be rejected. From a geriatrics point of view, multiple payers complicate life for the frail and beleaguered individual and family. The history of private insurance sold to the elderly is replete with signs of exploitation. To design a public program with financial gaps, or user fees, is an invitation to private insurers to fill the breach. But their cost for covering the gaps will exceed what a fuller public program would have cost. Medigap is an example that needs no duplication.

Private Insurance Is Chancy

The weaknesses of private insurance were discussed in Chapter Six. What may need emphasis here is that this private insurance is experimental, of questionable long-range stability, and is socially inefficient.

Private insurance offers little to build on. Some 60 to 65 cents of every premium dollar goes for overhead: sales and advertising, commissions, and so on. Part of the justification for withholding 40 cents from benefits is that large risks are taken. Insurers need reserves against adverse selection. They will also exclude people with certain preexisting conditions.

The costs of private insurance are high enough to make it unlikely that most people in old age will have coverage. Nor, because of the inflation factor, will those having the insurance be appreciably relieved of nursing home expenses. The Medicaid program probably will not be relieved of much of its burdens by private insurance. Private insurance is over its head in long-term care. And it is not cost-effective in long-term care.

A Foundation to Build On

What are the strengths to build on?

Social Insurance and State Experience

The nation can build on state experience in long-term care administration and federal experience with social insurance. The delivery of services will be in the hands of private or public sector organizations, including not-for-profit as well as for-profit entities. This pattern is found in some of the proposals discussed in Chapter Seven. It fits with the recommendations of the Pepper Commission, approved overwhelmingly by a bipartisan panel of commissioners. The panel, however, left small roles for private insurance and Medicaid in supporting long-term care in nursing homes.

Social insurance, in our view, answers better than any other form of financing the needs of long-term care and the protection of the middle class from impoverishment. Being compulsory, it establishes the largest pool of payers and users, has a relatively low overhead, and yields far better financial stability over the long run than smaller pools in private insurance.

There is no adverse selection to worry about, since coverage as well as payment is universal. Nor are there any games to be played with tests of assets and income and a "spend down."

The Question of Compulsion

Social insurance is universal because it is compulsory. This approach responds to long-term care as a necessity of modern life. We all have to have it, not only for ourselves but also for our families. It is not fair to those who save that those who could but do not save become public assistance recipients at taxpayer expense.

Through Medicare, our society compels people to contribute over their working lives to hospital insurance in old age. Never for a moment do we view this insurance as an unconscionable use of taxes to protect legacies. Why do we protect the victim of a heart attack, rich or poor, from the costs of acute care and not the victim of Alzheimer's disease, rich or poor, from the costs of long-term care?

Right or Privilege?

The explanation lies with the thinking of private insurance, which is market based. Some critics say this country has never decided one way or the other about access to health care as a right or a good to be bought in the marketplace. Would a market advocate agree to withhold life-saving services just because someone cannot pay? We do not think so.

Access to acute care or long-term care should *not* be conditioned on ability to pay or proof of poverty. For those who object to having health care as a simple human right, there is the American tradition of an earned right. All who contribute should benefit, whether rich or poor. This is not only equitable but good politics. The rich and poor are not set against one another, which would be the case if the rich were excluded by means testing. Franklin Roosevelt saw the political strength of universal benefits based on earned right and would not have denied social security even to the economic royalists he attacked.

It is no more fair to deny social insurance benefits to a rich person than it would be to deny that person the benefits of a fire insurance policy because of financial status.

The principles of social insurance now need to be applied to long-term care, making it an entitlement just as hospital insurance and social security old-age and disability benefits are earned entitlements. These are as much an expression of people taking responsibility for themselves as an investment in a tax-favored individual retirement account through a mutual fund is.

Insurance Thinking Versus Health Thinking

The problems we have shown with Medicare is that it originated in insurance thinking, replete with deductibles, coinsurance, and exclusions of preventive and long-term care services. It focuses on protection against acute care costs. The nursing home was attached to this model and transformed into a junior hospital. Home health care was a posthospital convalescence benefit. Long-term care — also known as custodial care — was a prohibited expense. What Medicare did not do, à la private insurance, was to exclude people with preexisting conditions.

It is now time to break barriers and open Medicare more fully to younger adults and dependent children.

Universal Coverage

The advantages of universal coverage, comprehensive benefits, and social or public insurance can be outlined briefly:

- *For individuals and families:* a user-friendly system; they no longer need to deal with a maze of entry points and eligibility requirements to obtain services; benefits and delivery methods are understandable; users have the help of a care coordinator; what helps older members of a family also helps younger members, and the reverse is true; no exclusion for preexisting conditions; the benefit is portable from job to job
- *For employers:* assistance to employees, facilitating their productivity; relief from pressure to provide a costly addition to fringe benefits

- *For provider organizations:* relief from multiple, duplicative, and inconsistent statutory and regulatory requirements of various agencies, micromanagement, and paperwork; systematizing permits flexibility (and experimentation) in service design and delivery based on results, cost efficiency, and local conditions; stable financing makes systems building possible
- *For home attendants:* the development of stable careers for homemakers and other paraprofessional personnel, including training and upward mobility based on accomplishment and skill; for physicians and nurses, a basis for the proper practice of geriatrics in various surroundings and through health and social service teamwork
- *For primary care practitioners:* a payment policy recognizing geriatric assessment, the special conditions of service to the very old in the office, home, nursing home, hospital, and elsewhere, and the need for teamwork among practitioners of many disciplines; a system that supports primary care with physicians trained in geriatrics, geriatric nurse practitioners, physician assistants, social workers, and care coordinators
- *For system organizers:* tools to achieve efficiency in managing long-term care and other resources (for example, data acquisition for policy and program decisions and utilization controls, including the study of sample populations over the years to determine effects of services on health)
- *For federal and state governments:* relief of pressures on Medicaid now and in the future, with savings applicable to federal and state deficits

Structuring a Long-Term Care Program

Building the program for long-term care security will be a complex undertaking. Parts already exist. The program will have to be built over the years as an essential part of the new American health care system, starting now to be well developed for the oncoming baby-boom cohort. The program should have consumer input in its administration and a definite schedule for implementing benefits and developing the personnel to deliver them. This can be carried off if the American people support a comprehensive approach strongly enough to overcome our legislative tendencies for piecemeal action.

The key recommendations for long-term care security include the following:

1. Long-term care policies should be integrated with reforms in the organization and financing of acute care and other health services. This should make it possible for various kinds of service organizations to combine to furnish a full continuum of care under payment and eligibility policies unbiased against categories of patients or service.
2. These policies may be implemented through national health insurance based wholly on a government program or a mixture of mandated job-based benefits covering the working population and an expanded Medicare covering all others. The Medicare component could cover long-term care for everyone as well as other health benefits for those not covered in the job-based program.
3. For purposes of buffering federal power, administration of all national health insurance — or the long-term care portion alone — could be lodged in a federally chartered corporation — a public utility having a nonpartisan board of governors advised by a national council of users, payers, and providers. The utility would set the rules for all payers. The utility would conduct research on service arrangements to determine effectiveness and efficiency.
4. The reforms would eliminate Medicaid. States that have had valuable experience with long-term care development would be delegated administration of long-term care benefits, as indicated by the Pepper Commission plan. The long-term care program developed and operated by the state under federal standards would make payments. Under contract, local public or voluntary nonprofit agencies would conduct assessments, care planning, and service coordination and monitoring. Certified nonprofit and for-profit organizations would provide services. Liaison between health and housing, transportation, and other nonhealth activities would be encouraged.
5. Funds will be needed to expedite the development of community-based and other long-term care service organiza-

tions. Funds also would be needed to promote construction of assisted-care and other residential facilities. Loans
could be made from accumulations in the main social security trust fund and repaid with interest from service payments. Loans would be justified as contributing to the goals
of social security.

6.   To promote quality of the systems and the care they give,
the following actions would be taken:

a.   Increased federal and state grants for the geriatrics education of physicians, nurses, administrators, and other
professional and semiprofessional workers.

b.   Incorporating in the local care-planning agency an advisory council of system users of all ages and payers
(for example, older persons in the community and
nursing home, wage earners of all ages, and employers). The councils would make studies and receive for
evaluation the comments, suggestions, and complaints
of system users and payers.

c.   Expanding grants under the Older Americans Act to
develop volunteer services in the community, including transportation, meals-on-wheels, friendly visiting,
and chore services.

7.   To help control costs and improve the effectiveness and
efficiency of services, research on the delivery, organization,
and outcomes of services and technology would be conducted.

Teaching the Users

The public should be informed about the entry points, the benefits, and their rights under the program to make complaints
and appeals. Consumers should be recruited to form advisory
groups to the local long-term care program. Since the program
depends on both paid and volunteer services, strong community support and involvement in the program are vital. The
program should furnish technical assistance to communities that
want to develop volunteer services for friendly visiting, transportation, telephone assurance, and other efforts.

The program would teach care procedures to family members and support groups. Able and willing family members could be taught to administer injections, to give cardiopulmonary resuscitation, and to carry out other procedures. There would be a twenty-four-hour telephone number to call for advice on what to do in a crisis.

Individuals would be referred to the long-term care program from physician offices, hospitals, and other places of health and social service. Every telephone book would carry a number for access to the program. Broadcast and cable television channels would carry information about access to the program as well as discussions on how to handle programs connected with long-term care.

The program also would send representatives to public and private schools as well as employment sites to educate about long-term care. They would explain how people of all ages may assist the disabled through volunteer and other efforts.

Training Practitioners and Administrators

The federal and state governments, in concert with private organizations, will need to carry out a long-term plan for developing the personnel to operate the program. One step is to promote training in geriatrics among professionals, notably physicians, nurses, social workers, and therapists. Every medical student and resident should be trained in geriatrics. All professional schools should rotate students through various sites of care — in the institution, in the community, and at home. Moving medical schools in this direction will require strong financial incentives. At the same time, the payment methods under the comprehensive national health insurance system should ensure fair compensation for geriatrics.

Personal Care Workers. A particular effort would be made to train personal care workers, a title that would include home health aides, homemakers, and aides in nursing homes. A qualified personal care worker could work in any home or institutional setting. A career pathway should be established to recognize skills and supervisory talent. Studies should be done to establish fair pay and benefits for these workers. Efforts in long-term care should be recognized as being on a par with work in a hospital.

Care Coordinators. Pivotal in the new systems will be care coordinators. They must gain the trust of families and individuals as well as professional practitioners and administrators. The care coordinator is both an advocate of the system user and a conservator of the system's resources — a potential conflict of interest. Perhaps one of the best ways to maintain public confidence is to locate care coordinators in agencies with heavy public representation on their governing boards. Although social workers and nurses often are care coordinators, individuals with good general educations can be trained to do the tasks. The State of Oregon has a one-month program of formal training followed up by training on the job. These coordinators are said to be well accepted by the public.

The Patient as Supervisor

The national program should also build on experience and concepts in the disability field by giving competent and willing patients the authority to supervise their own care at home. This may extend to hiring and firing personal care workers, with the overall situation supervised by care coordinators.

Care Innovations

The program should experiment with new methods of care and organization, with consideration given to the development of outcome-based standards of service and payment. For example, in carrying out the plan of care for an individual, full payment would be made if objectives are completely achieved on schedule, and partial payment if not. Such a system would reward methods of care that are found to prevent complications.

Facilitative Environments

In promoting independence, the new program should emphasize making the home environment as usable and safe as possible for the disabled individual. It should also collaborate with housing organizations to establish regular service offices where frail or disabled individuals were clustered. For example, a nurse and social worker might be located in an office near several housing projects with many frail and disabled persons. This kind of arrangement, being applied on a wide scale in Japan under its ten-year plan of long-term care development, has worked successfully in American congregate housing demonstrations. The long-term care program could collaborate with housing programs in orienting managers and guards to problems of the frail and disabled. The housing programs could involve not only new construction but also retrofitting, rehabilitation, and provision for shared living arrangements.

Vertical Integration of Providers

Incentives could be provided for diverse facilities — such as HMOs, hospitals, nursing homes, home care agencies, adult day-care facilities, and assisted housing facilities — to work together to achieve continuums of care. Programs should be encouraged to experiment with innovative services and clusters of services to improve the effectiveness and patient acceptability of long-term care. And programs that support constructing nursing homes, adult day care, and other facilities in accord with local population needs for institutional and noninstitutional care are required.

In the Community, at the Job

The new program also should promote the development of adult day-care centers and other places where its beneficiaries could receive needed services, paid and volunteered. Business and labor unions may contribute through employee assistance programs to the development of these centers and volunteer groups. Continuing care retirement communities should divert income to benefits other than long-term care.

Transportation

To get the frail and disabled to outpatient clinics for medical, nursing, rehabilitative, and other services, the program should pay for transportation or help communities develop their own transportation networks for these beneficiaries.

The Costs

In their pacesetting study, *Caring for the Disabled Elderly: Who Will Pay?* Alice M. Rivlin and Joshua M. Wiener (1988, p. 238) phrase the economics of the long-term care debate in this way: "The question is not whether spending for long-term care will rise, but by whom these costs will be borne. Will they be borne largely by people unlucky enough to need expensive care, or will they be borne by society more broadly? And how will the costs be divided between the public and private sectors?"

In the Rivlin-Wiener analysis, long-term care in 2016–2020 — without any changes in current policy — would cost $120 billion a year, of which Medicaid would pay $48.6 billion and Medicare $9.3 billion, other payers $7.2 billion, and patients and families $54.9 billion.

A full public program of long-term care would raise total spending to $157.2 billion, of which $124.7 million would be principally an expanded Medicare. The bulk of long-term care would move from Medicaid and out-of-pocket spending to the public insurance program. The system would spend $37 billion more than under the old pattern, but it would lessen the toll exacted by out-of-pocket spending and premiums.

The Pepper Commission, which mixes user fees and liberalized Medicaid with social insurance, estimated $42.5 billion a year at program maturity (in 1990 dollars). This amount equals 5 percent of total spending for personal health care in the United States; it is half or less of one year's health care inflation.

Earmarked Taxes

As proposed by Rivlin and Wiener, a comprehensive program could be funded by a payroll tax plus current public spending for long-term care, as proposed in a Brookings Institution study. The payroll tax would be about 1.6 percent each for employer and employee from now through 2020. For $30,000-a-year earners, the tax works out to $240 each annually for employers and employees, or less than $5 a week from an individual employee's pocket.

Cutting Waste

If the United States could eliminate waste in health care, the savings should be more than enough to finance the Pepper Commission plan without new taxes. With 1,500 insurance companies and thousands of health policies and variations in benefits, the payment paperwork is costly as well as confusing. Using the Canadian system as a framework, an estimated $65 billion could be saved in the United States under simplified administration and uniform benefits. The magnitude of waste is suggested also by the National Leadership Coalition for Health Care Reform, whose honorary co-chairs are former Presidents Carter and Ford. The coalition asserts that its form of national health insurance would cut annual health care costs by more than $600 billion by the end of the 1990s compared to what an unreformed system is expected to cost.

Social Security Overcollections

Another source of funds to develop long-term care lies in the Social Security System. Currently, it is building up an enormous trust fund to help pay for the baby-boom retirements. An estimated $8 trillion will be accumulated before payouts exceed income in the first quarter of the twenty-first century.

The accumulation was not designed for the baby-boom retirements. The Social Security Reform Commission in 1983 was faced with a serious immediate shortage of funds for old-age and survivors' insurance. In adopting a schedule of payroll tax increases to meet that need, the commission recognized that by the early 1990s, the schedule should be reconsidered, because the system would then be well stabilized. That reconsideration has not happened.

Amassing a huge trust fund is not the only way to provide for the baby boomers. Assuming a thriving U.S. economy over the long term, the current schedule could be reduced and the baby-boom retirees could be financed through small periodic changes in the payroll tax rate.

Senator Daniel Patrick Moynihan (D-N.Y.) has proposed returning the current "overcollections" to the taxpayers by reducing the tax rate. But they could be returned in the form of long-term care coverage instead. A portion of the trust fund accumulations or a portion of the current tax rate also might be assigned to capitalizing the service organizations and facilities needed in long-term care systems as well as to paying for the services. Protection against impoverishment, the rationale for adding Medicare to the Social Security System, also justifies covering long-term care under social insurance.

Other Tax Options

There are other tax options besides additional payroll taxes earmarked for long-term care. An increase in the rate of tax on estates and gifts could be assigned to long-term care. The new protections would help conserve legacies.

In short, the financing of long-term care is not an insuperable barrier.

Phasing in the Benefits

In 1965–66, Medicare could be introduced relatively quickly because the infrastructure (providers and insurance administration) was already in place. The administrative base for a national long-term care program exists only partially. It is found in state Medicaid and Older Americans Act programs and in Medicare's use of state health departments to check on nursing homes, home health agencies, and other providers. In a few states, the infrastructure is relatively well developed for community-based as well as nursing home care.

The Pepper Commission proposed a four-year implementation program, as follows (with cost in 1990 dollars): In year 1 ($10.8 billion), the home and community-based care program would start, providing up to 200 hours per person per year. In year 2 ($25.0 billion), the three-month nursing home benefit under social insurance would begin; coverage of longer stays under a Medicaid-type program would begin, and reform of nursing home payment rates would be introduced. In year 3 ($32.8 billion), the home and community-based care benefit would expand to 400 hours. Year 4 ($42.8 billion) would see full implementation of the home and community-based program and further improvements in nursing home payment rates.

Minimally, a first phase should focus on the very old and provide assessment, care planning, and care coordination. This pattern was described in New York's EISEP program (Chapter Four). A first phase in a broader approach might include, like the Pepper Commission plan, provision of an amount of home care. From the very beginning, some investment should be made in training of personnel, including administrators, and public education in the nature of long-term care and self-help. The needs of younger adults and children should be studied so that services and assessment methods are appropriate.

Whatever period is chosen for phasing, the objectives should not be in doubt. Given legislation that sets out principles, goals, and rough timetables, detailed plans could be developed with advice from a network of national and regional groups of providers, payers, educators, volunteers, and potential users.

Beyond Medicare

Medicare evolved from the defeat of national health insurance more than forty years ago. It was devised to cover individuals left out of mainstream job-based insurance coverage. Unfortunately, though meant chiefly for elders, Medicare was not designed for geriatrics. Medicare has fallen behind the demographics: we have a rapidly growing population of very old people. The quest for a fair, affordable, and secure long-term care policy is part of the adaptation of our institutions and life-styles to the opportunities and needs posed by long lifetimes. The growing population of AIDS victims is a major long-term care challenge.

Medicare was considered by national health insurance advocates as a demonstration that a government health insurance program could work at least as well as conventional private insurance at its best. Now, as that private system falters, the United States may be ready to move beyond Medicare.

The problems of covering long-term care are not only the problems of the old or the disabled. Nor are these problems confined to the portion of our economy covering health and social services. The problems affect us all because of the evolving conditions of life summed up in the word *longevity*. "The subject of our lunchtime conversations has shifted," columnist Ellen Goodman has noted. "Once they leaned heavily toward pediatrics. Now they include geriatrics." People live longer, and more of them reach old age. Our institutions—not just health care institutions—are lagging behind the longevity curve. The design of housing, automobiles, appliances, and fine-print contract forms must be reconsidered to accommodate people when they are disabled as well as when they are hale and hearty. Life cycle fairness demands it, or else we pay dearly in loss of dignity and relative independence. People should have the freedom of "aging in place," of directing their own care, of continuing to contribute to family, society, and self for as long as they are able.

Our institutions have to meet the later life cycle half way. Those institutions that manage to raise barriers in proportion to age and disability—such as in the fields of health insurance and public assistance—are ready for terminal care and a curt goodbye.

There are those who claim that the old are exploiting the young. Intergenerational equity is among the most divisive concepts in our society. It is used in attacks on social security, ignoring that program's life cycle applications; social security benefits are received by two million children of deceased or disabled workers. From a family perspective, a benefit received by a member at one stage of the life cycle has positive effects on other members.

Nonetheless, intergenerational equity arguments are used against financing long-term care benefits. On the issue of whether America can afford long-term care, the answer may not lie with intergenerational equity nearly as much as with the ancient war of rich and poor and who pays their fair share of taxes (Lekach- man, 1987).

Whether longevity is triumph or burden depends on how society — as well as individuals — uses resources. The kneeling bus, the van for wheelchair patients, building entrance ramps, traffic lights with longer intervals, highways with bigger signs and longer exit lanes, and vision and hearing aids represent an evolving accommodation, a continuing welcome of people with chronic disabilities to the mainstreams of American life. The finest accommodation — a gift of all of us to ourselves and fam- ilies — is the security of knowing that we never outlive our access to humane and skillful long-term care.

REFERENCES

Ball, R. M. *Because We're All in This Together: The Case for a National Long-Term Care Insurance Policy.* Washington, D.C.: Families USA, 1989.

Brody, J. A., and Persky, V. A. "Epidemiology and Demographics." In W. B. Abrams and R. Berkow (eds.), *The Merck Manual of Geriatrics.* Rahway, N.J.: Merck Sharp & Dohme Research Laboratories, 1990.

Butler, R. N. *Why Survive? Being Old in America.* New York: HarperCollins, 1975.

Butler, R. N., and Gleason, H. P. (eds.). *Productive Aging: Enhancing Vitality in Later Life.* New York: Springer, 1985.

Commonwealth Fund Commission on Elderly People Living Alone. *Help at Home: Long-Term Care Assistance for Impaired Elderly People.* Baltimore, Md.: Commonwealth Fund Commission on Elderly People Living Alone, 1989.

Congressional Budget Office. *Policy Choices for Long-Term Care.* Washington, D.C.: Congressional Budget Office, 1991.

Davis, K. "Response to Robert E. Patricelli." In Institute of Medicine, *Providing Universal and Affordable Health Care.* Washington, D.C.: National Academy of Sciences, 1989.

DelPonte, P. "Meeting the Medical Needs of the Senior Boom: The National Shortage of Geriatricians." *Alliance for Aging Research,* Apr. 1992.

Densen, P. M. *Tracing the Elderly Through the Health Care System:*

An Update. Rockville, Md.: Agency for Health Care Policy and Research, 1991.

Doty, P., Liu, K., Manton, K., and Harahan, M. "Patterns of Medicaid 'Spend Down' Associated with Long-Term Care." Paper presented at the meeting of the Gerontological Society of America, Minneapolis, Nov. 1989.

Executive Office on Aging, Office of the Governor, State of Hawaii. *Financing Long-Term Care: A Report to the Hawaii State Legislature.* Honolulu: Executive Office on Aging, Office of the Governor, State of Hawaii, 1991.

Fineman, L. *Summary Paper: Community Care System for the Elderly in Manitoba, Canada.* Winnipeg, Manitoba: Office of Home Care, 1992.

Fox, K. S. "Assessing Home Care Policy and Its Effect on the Elderly." *Blueprint* (newsletter of the United Hospital Fund of New York), Spring/Summer 1989.

General Accounting Office. *Long-Term Care: Projected Needs of the Aging Baby Boom Generation.* Document no. GAO/HRD-91-86. Washington, D.C.: General Accounting Office, 1991.

General Accounting Office. *Long-Term Care Insurance: Actions Needed to Reduce Risks to Consumers.* Document no. GAO/HRD-92-66. Washington, D.C.: General Accounting Office, 1992.

Gompertz, B. "On the Nature of the Function Expressive of the Law of Human Mortality, and on a New Mode of Determining the Value of Life Contingencies." *Philosophical Transactions of the Royal Society,* 1825, *115,* 513.

Hunt, T. E. "Rehabilitation of the Elderly." In W. Reichel (ed.), *The Geriatric Patient.* New York: HP Publishing, 1978.

Institute of Medicine. *America's Aging: Health in an Older Society.* Washington, D.C.: National Research Council, 1985.

Joint American Medical Association/American Nurses Association Task Force to Address the Improvement of Health Care of the Aged Chronically Ill. *Report.* Kansas City, Mo.: Joint American Medical Association/American Nurses Association Task Force to Address the Improvement of Health Care of the Aged Chronically Ill, 1983.

Kane, R. A., and Kane, R. L. *Long-Term Care: Principles, Programs, and Policies.* New York: Springer, 1987.

Kane, R. L., and others. *Geriatrics in the United States: Manpower Projections and Training Considerations.* Santa Monica, Calif.: Rand Corporation, 1980.

Kemper, P., and Murtaugh, C. "Lifetime Use of Nursing Home Care." *New England Journal of Medicine,* 1991, *324* (1), 595–600.

Lekachman, R. "A Mystery Solved." *New Leader,* Oct. 5, 1987, pp. 18–20.

Leutz, W., and others. *Adding Long-Term Care to Medicine: The Social HMO Experience.* Waltham, Mass.: Bigel Institute, Heller School, Brandeis University, 1990.

Levit, K. R., Lazenby, H. C., Cowan, C. A., and Letsch, S. W. "National Health Expenditures, by Type of Expenditure and Source of Funds." *Health Care Financing Review,* 1991, *13*(1), 29–54.

McConnell, S. "Public Opinion on Long-Term Care: A Review of National Opinion Surveys." *Proceedings of the Long-Term Care Committee of the Commonwealth Fund Commission on Elderly People Living Alone.* Background Papers Series, no. 11. Baltimore, Md.: Commonwealth Fund Commission, 1988.

Maddox, G. L., and Manton, K. G. "Hospitals: The DRG System." In K. C. Eisdorfer, D. A. Kessler, and A. N. Spector (eds.), *Caring for the Elderly: Reshaping Health Policy.* Baltimore, Md.: Johns Hopkins University Press, 1989.

Manitoba Health Department. *Quality Health for Manitobans: The Action Plan.* Winnipeg, Manitoba, Canada: Manitoba Health Department, 1992.

Moloney, T. W. *Overview: The Commission as a Model.* New York: The Commission on Elderly Living Alone, 1987.

Muller, C., Fahs, M. C., and Schechter, M. "Primary Medical Care for Elderly Patients: Parts I and II." *Journal of Community Health,* 1989, *14*(2), 79–98.

National Center for Health Statistics. "Current Estimates from the National Health Interview Survey, 1989." *Vital and Health Statistics,* Oct. 1990, series 10, no. 176.

National Chronic Care Consortium. *The NCC Today: Where We Are and Where We Are Going.* Bloomington, Minn.: National Chronic Care Consortium, 1993.

National Institute on Aging. *Personnel for Health Needs of the Elderly*

Through Year 2020. Report to Congress. Washington, D.C.:
U.S. Department of Health and Human Services, 1987.

Pallan, P. "Serving Elderly Patients: The Benefits of Integrated
Long-Term Care in British Columbia." In A. Bennett and
O. Adams (eds.), *Looking North for Health: What We Can Learn
from Canada's Health Care System.* San Francisco: Jossey-Bass,
1993.

Paone, D. Quoted in "Geriatric Services Grow." *Hospitals,* Jan.
5, 1993, p. 32.

Pepper Commission. *A Call for Action.* Final report. Washington, D.C.: Government Printing Office, 1990.

Pfeiffer, E. "The Need for Faculty Development in Geriatric
Medicine." *Journal of the American Geriatrics Society,* 1977, *25,*
490–491.

Polniaszek, S. E. *Long-Term Care: A Dollar and Sense Guide.* (Rev.
ed.) Washington, D.C.: United Seniors Health Cooperative,
1992.

Polniaszek, S. E., and Firman, J. P. *Long-Term Care Insurance:
A Professional's Guide to Selecting Policies.* Washington, D.C.:
United Seniors Health Cooperative, 1991.

Productive Aging News. "Geriatrics: The Urgent Need for Investment." June 1992, pp. 1–3.

Program Resources Department, American Association of Retired Persons, and U.S. Administration on Aging. *A Profile
of Older Americans.* Washington, D.C.: Program Resources
Department, American Association of Retired Persons, and
U.S. Administration on Aging, 1991.

Public Policy Institute, American Association of Retired Persons. *Changing Needs for Long-Term Care: A Chartbook.* Washington, D.C.: American Association of Retired Persons, 1989.

Reilly, T. W., Clauser, S. B., and Baugh, D. K. "Trends in
Medicaid Payments and Utilization, 1975–1989." *Health Care
Financing Review* (1990 Annual Supplement).

Rice, D. P. "Introduction." *Generations,* 1985, *9*(4), 6.

Rice, T. "The Use, Cost, and Economic Burden of Nursing-
Home Care in 1985." *Medical Care,* 1989, *27*(12), 1133–1147.

Riley, M. W., Ory, M. G., and Zablotsky, D. (eds.). *AIDS
in an Aging Society: What We Need to Know.* New York: Springer,
1989.

Rivlin, A. M., and Wiener, J. M. *Caring for the Disabled Elderly: Who Will Pay?* Washington, D.C.: Brookings Institution, 1988.

Rossman, I. "Options for Care of the Aged Sick." In W. Reichel (ed.), *The Geriatric Patient.* New York: HP Publishing, 1978.

Scanlon, W. J. *Long-Term Care: Economic Impacts and Financing Dilemmas.* New York: National Health Council, 1990.

Schneider, E. L., and Guralnik, J. M. "The Aging of America: Impact on Health Care Costs." *Journal of the American Medical Association,* 1990, *263*(17), 2335–2339.

Select Committee on Aging, U.S. House of Representatives. *Exploding the Myths: Caregiving in America.* Washington, D.C.: Government Printing Office, 1987.

Simon-Rusinowitz, L. *Personal Assistance Services for the Elderly Under Medicaid: Examining Cost-Quality Trade-Offs.* Issue Brief no. 582. Washington, D.C.: National Health Policy Forum, 1991.

Special Committee on Aging, U.S. Senate. *Developments in Aging: 1985.* Vol. 3. Washington, D.C.: Government Printing Office, 1986.

Special Committee on Aging, U.S. Senate. *Developments in Aging: 1987.* Vol. 3. Washington, D.C.: Government Printing Office, 1988.

Special Committee on Aging, U.S. Senate. *Aging America.* Washington, D.C.: Government Printing Office, 1989.

Stone, R., Cafferata, G. L., and Sangl, J. *Caregivers of the Frail Elderly: A National Profile.* Washington, D.C.: U.S. Department of Health and Human Services, 1986.

Stone, R., and Kemper, P. "Spouses and Children of Disabled Elders: How Large a Constituency for Long-Term Care Reform?" *Milbank Quarterly,* 1989, *67,* 3–4. Unpublished appendix.

Task Force on Long-Term Health Care Policies, U.S. Department of Health and Human Services. *Report to Congress and the Secretary.* Washington, D.C.: U.S. Department of Health and Human Services, 1988.

Tilly, J., and Stucki, B. R. *International Perspectives on Long-Term Care Reform in the United States.* Washington, D.C.: Public Policy Institute, American Association of Retired Persons, 1991.

U.S. Bureau of the Census. "Estimates of the Population of the

United States, by Single Years of Age, Color, and Sex: 1900 to 1959." *Current Population Reports,* July 1965, series P-25, no. 311.

U.S. Bureau of the Census. "Marital Status and Living Arrangements: March 1989." *Current Population Reports,* June 1990b, series P-20, no. 445.

U.S. Bureau of the Census. "Projections of the Population of the United States, by Age, Sex, and Race: 1988 to 2080," by G. Spencer. *Current Population Reports,* Jan. 1989, series P-25, no. 1018.

U.S. Bureau of the Census. *Statistical Abstract of the United States, 1987.* Washington, D.C.: Government Printing Office, 1987.

U.S. Bureau of the Census. *Statistical Abstract of the United States, 1992.* Washington, D.C.: Government Printing Office, 1992.

U.S. Bureau of the Census. "U.S. Population Estimates, by Age, Sex, Race, and Hispanic Origin: 1989," by F. W. Hollman. *Current Population Reports,* Mar. 1990a, series P-25, no. 1057.

Varner, T. *Catastrophic Health Care for Older Americans: The Issue and Its Implications for Policy Development.* Washington, D.C.: American Association of Retired Persons, 1987.

Waldo, D. R., and Lazenby, H. C. "Demographic Characteristics and Health Care Expenditures by Age in the United States, 1977–1984." *Health Care Financing Review,* 1984, *6*(1), 1–29.

Waldo, D. R., Sonnefeld, S. T., McKusick, D. R., and Arnett, R. H. III. "Health Care Expenditures by Age Group, 1977 and 1987." *Health Care Financing Review,* 1989, *10*(4), 111–120.

Wiener, J. M., and Hanley, R. J. "The Connecticut Model for Financing Long-Term Care: A Limited Partnership?" *Journal of the American Geriatrics Society,* 1992, *40*(10), 1069–1072.

INDEX